Just Enough Healthcare

Siv Raman

This page left intentionally blank

Table of Contents

COPYRIGHTS AND ATTRIBUTIONS

Author contact information
Dr. Sivakumaran "Siv" Raman
Twitter: @RamanSiv (https://twitter.com/ramansiv)

Credits
Cover Art: Dr. Saurabh Sheel
Proofreading: Dr. Tarakad Subbarama Raman

Publishing History
July-2020 First Edition

Copyright Details
Copyright © 2020 Sivakumaran Raman

Book-writing tools
This book was written using LibreOffice 6.0 on a desktop computer running Ubuntu Linux 18.04. GIMP 2.10 was used for creating the cover and for photo editing. Calibre 4.20 was used to create and edit the e-book version of the text.

DEDICATION

To my loving wife and children, who motivated me to write this book, and to my parents, who have always been there for me.

ACKNOWLEDGMENTS

I am grateful to my father, Dr. Tarakad Subbarama Raman, for proofreading this book. My sincere appreciation to my friend and medical-college classmate, Dr. Saurabh Sheel, for creating the artwork for the book cover. My thanks to the developers that made the open-source tools Linux, LibreOffice, GIMP, and Calibre – all of which I used to create this book. Lastly, I want to thank my family for their continued love and support.

This page left intentionally blank

INTRODUCTION

Healthcare is one of the largest sectors of the US economy. Per 2017 figures, US healthcare spending of $3.5 trillion[1] was 18 percent of the country's Gross Domestic Product (GDP). The US *Health Care and Social Assistance* sector[2] alone employed about 19 million individuals at the end of 2016. The constituents of this sector do not include health insurance companies, Health Information Technology companies, and related entities. Therefore, the true number of healthcare-industry employees is likely to be significantly higher.

An intriguing thing about the healthcare industry is how siloed the employees are in the work they perform. I have met IT professionals who have worked for years in a health insurance firm that do not understand how a physician arrives at a diagnosis or what the Explanation of Benefits (EOB) mailed to them by the health plan contains. Similarly, I have met practicing physicians who have no clue what terms like Guaranteed Issue, Community Rating, and Medical Cost/Loss Ratio mean.

This is what prompted me to write this book: *a pick-up-and-read-through introduction to all things healthcare.* This is a primer text that can be used to get a broad overview of the US Healthcare system in just a single day. This book seeks to become *the* first resource for anyone who wants to get an understanding of US healthcare without spending 6 months doing so. No attempt is made to go into the full detail of the topics presented. However, my hope is that readers who complete the book will achieve a framework-level understanding of healthcare and develop the ability to seek out more detailed information on topics of interest to them.

All through this book, I use the term "healthcare" instead of "health care" or the hyphenated "health-care", because I feel that the single-word term conveys the meaning best.

BASTIAT'S "BROKEN WINDOW" PARABLE APPLIED TO HEALTHCARE (IT SHOULD NOT BE!)

Why economic arguments sound inhumane

when applied to healthcare!

Applying economic theory to healthcare is fraught with danger, mainly because healthcare goods and services are unlike other goods and services in the economy. Very few other goods and services have the power to affect and extend life. Also, many if not all modern societies have come to see healthcare as a right (even if it is not considered a *natural right* since it costs money to provide healthcare), and thus do not want economic considerations to be used to decide who gets it and how much. Thus, applying economic constraints and free-market thinking to healthcare sometimes results in what are viewed as heartless solutions. I present an unsympathetic example here of applying the Broken Window parable of economics to healthcare as a cautionary lesson.

Frédéric Bastiat, a French economist, used the parable of the broken window[3] to illustrate that the breaking of a window and the subsequent expenditure of money to fix it does not generate economic growth or a net benefit to society. In other words, resources used to repair or replace damaged or destroyed capital do not spur economic growth. Several things about the broken-window parable seem analogous to the healthcare system in America. Chronically sick individuals who are not able to contribute to economic activity can be crudely considered (from a purely economic and clearly heartless perspective) the human equivalents of broken windows. This is even more so when we are talking about people with diseases like type 2 diabetes and heart disease that could have been prevented through factors like diet and exercise. You can see how dehumanizing this is towards patients and the provision of healthcare - I offer this imperfect analogy only to illustrate how applying *purely* economic arguments to healthcare, without human and moral considerations, leads to the degrading branding of sick people as burdens on society.

The other piece of information that is critical to understand is that 20% of the US population drives 80% of the healthcare expenditure.[4] In fact, 5% of the population drives 50% of the healthcare expenditure!

Also, a large percentage of the medical expenditure related to a person occurs in the last few years of life.[5] Topping this off is the fact that in a number of US states, the largest employer is a health system.[6]

Even taking into account that healthcare is a labor-intensive industry, this still seems to drive towards the cold-hearted economic argument that the country is spending trillions to treat sick people, many of whom could have avoided getting sick in the first place (with proper preventative care and lifestyle modifications). Expressed in cold economic terms, there is a huge opportunity cost of all this spending on healthcare. Are we sacrificing economic growth and a net-benefit to society to keep investing so much in medical care? In fact, extrapolating the Bastiat "Broken Window" fallacy further, a lot of the resources expended in replacing/repairing damaged human capital (through the provision of healthcare services) does not actually lead to societal/economic growth, since the human capital was not contributing to economic activity in the first place. In many cases, millions and billions are being spent on the (again uncompassionate) economic equivalent of working on a vintage, non-working car that cannot be used for transportation.

Thus, in a way, the grand (political, ethical, and social) debate becomes:

(1) Do we uphold our belief in unbounded healthcare as a human right by making sure everyone gets at least a bare minimum of essential care (i.e. the socialized healthcare solution that has been implemented in many other developed countries but usually includes some degree of rationing of care)?

or

(2) Do we treat healthcare as just another economic good/service and leave it up to the free market to decide who gets what and how much of?

That is a choice the American people will have to make soon. And cold economics alone cannot be the basis for this decision. Politics, ethics, and many other factors play into making these choices as a nation.

WHOM IS THIS BOOK FOR?

This book is for anyone interested in getting a wide-angle introduction to the healthcare system. The country-level focus is on the US but many parts of the text apply to healthcare in other countries as well. The target reader for the book could be an information technology, finance, or law professional with no clinical background working for a US healthcare company. Or it could even be a physician, nurse, or pharmacist working in a hospital or clinic who knows a lot about clinical practice but wants to understand the insurance, billing, and revenue side of healthcare. Another category of reader could be the offshore employee of a US healthcare corporation who wants to get an idea of the business of healthcare in America.

Healthcare is so vast in its scope that even those who have been working in the industry for years understand just their own sub-domains. And the hindrances to learning about other healthcare subject areas are numerous: steep learning curves, the unavailability of documented information, the wall of jargon, and the paucity of time.

This book aims to address all of these obstacles to getting a holistic understanding of the healthcare industry. After finishing this book, the reader will be enriched with a broad working understanding of the US healthcare system. The book does not seek to go deep into the weeds of the topics being discussed, as that would require an encyclopedia-size text. It does not attempt to detail, examine, and analyze. Instead, the aim is to *simplify* for *clarity* of *understanding*. The book's goal is to get the reader up and running within a short period of time with a practical understanding of the business and processes of healthcare. Since an understanding of the "business" is what separates good leaders from the rest, this book will help the reader become a better leader in their sub-domain of the healthcare industry.

1. THE PARTICIPANTS IN HEALTHCARE

Our journey to understand the healthcare industry starts with an examination of the major participants in it. These are:

- Providers
- Private Payers
- Members and Patients
- Life Science Companies
- Pharmacy Benefit Managers
- Government Entities including payers like Medicare

PROVIDERS

"Provider" is a generic term used to describe any person or entity that *provides* healthcare services. Therefore, the word can be applied to a physician, a nurse, a nurse practitioner, a physician assistant, a chiropractor, a pharmacist, a pharmacy, a hospital, a health system, an outpatient surgery center, a clinical laboratory facility, a medical clinic, and many other individuals and organizations.

Since providers are directly involved in the *provision* of healthcare, they are usually the individuals and entities that we come into contact with when we seek clinical services.

Hospitals

Hospitals are one of the most important kinds of organizational providers.[7] Hospitals are institutions or organizations that provide specialized care, usually involving patients admitted and staying at the facility for some length of time. Emergency rooms are usually part of hospital facilities from where incoming patients can be admitted as inpatients to the wards. Hospitals can be of many kinds: teaching, community, charitable, religiously-affiliated, not-for-profit, for-profit, etc. These classifications are not mutually exclusive.

PAYERS

"Payer" is a term used to describe the third-party payer-entities that ultimately take on the financial risk of covering the costs (i.e. paying for) of medical care. Payers can be private health insurance companies but can also be government entities like Medicare and Medicaid. However, usually the term

payer is used to refer to a private payer instead of a government entity. The US is said to have a "third-party" payer system for healthcare since the patients/consumers who utilize healthcare services do not usually reimburse the providers directly. Instead, the payment is usually made by the health insurance company that has insured the consumers and assumed healthcare-services financial risk for them.

MEMBERS AND PATIENTS

The term "member" is used by a health insurance company (payer) to refer to an individual who is covered by a health insurance plan. The term "subscriber" usually refers to the primary member in whose name the health plan policy is created and sold. The dependents (usually family and relations) of the subscriber are all members of the health plan. Therefore, all subscribers are members but not all members are subscribers. The term "patient" is used for a person seeking healthcare services in a clinical setting. It is usually utilized by healthcare workers like physicians, nurses, and pharmacists. Therefore, all members are potential patients (if they seek healthcare services). However, not all patients are members. Patients who are not covered by a health insurance plan (uninsured individuals) are not considered to be members of any health plan.

LIFE SCIENCE COMPANIES

The term "life science company" is a catch-all for pharmaceutical companies, medical device companies, biotechnology companies, food processing companies, and related entities that create products and services that assist in the delivery of healthcare. Life science companies do not act directly as *providers*. But they provide a lot of the product-innovation and services that are ancillary to the delivery of effective healthcare.

PHARMACEUTICAL DISTRIBUTORS & PHARMACY BENEFIT MANAGERS

Pharmaceutical Distributors/Wholesalers are middlemen involved in the process of purchasing pharmaceutical products from pharmaceutical companies and selling them to entities like pharmacies, pharmacy benefit managers, and health plans. The interactions between all these entities are complex.

Pharmacy Benefit Managers or PBMs are the great mysteries of the healthcare world. Very few people understand the role they play and many are confused about why the health insurance company cannot play the role of the PBM. However, PBMs play a critical role in administering prescription drug programs for members of a health plan. PBMs facilitate pharmacy coverage for medications/prescriptions while helping to control drug costs. Per the American Pharmacists Association (AphA),[8] *"PBMs are primarily responsible for developing and maintaining the formulary, contracting with pharmacies, negotiating discounts and rebates with drug manufacturers, and processing and paying prescription drug claims. For the most part, they work with self-insured companies and government programs striving to maintain or reduce the pharmacy expenditures of the plan while concurrently trying to improve health care outcomes."*

Health insurance companies, employers purchasing health insurance for employees, government agencies, and many other entities contract with PBMs for delivering the pharmacy/medication part of the healthcare benefits to their members. If an employer or other purchaser of health insurance buys both the medical and pharmacy benefits from the health plan, it is known as a carve-in pharmacy arrangement. This is the most common case with fully-insured arrangements (which we will read about later). Even in a carve-in pharmacy arrangement, the health plan might engage the PBM for the pharmacy benefits administration. The other arrangement, a carve-out pharmacy, is when the insurance purchaser purchases medical benefits from the health plan but contracts directly with the PBM for pharmacy benefits. This is seen more commonly in self-insured arrangements (which is another concept we will read about later). PBMs help control drug costs by negotiating discounted prices on drugs (from retail pharmacies and manufacturers), managing medication utilization, and automating services. Thus, they play a vital role in the health system, at least when it comes to medications.

GOVERNMENT ENTITIES

US Federal and State governments directly pay for approximately half of the healthcare delivered in the country. In fact, some studies claim that taxpayers fund 64% of US healthcare.[9]

This might come as a surprise to many, especially since the US does not have government-run healthcare or a socialized medicine system. Medicare (government-funded healthcare for seniors and certain other special groups), Medicaid (US Federal and state funded healthcare for the indigent), and the Children's Health Insurance Program (CHIP) make up most of the government-funded healthcare in America.

EMPLOYERS

US employers who purchase and provide health insurance coverage for their employees together are major participants in the healthcare system. This is because almost 50% of the US population receives health insurance coverage from an employer. The US tax code also provides generous tax deductions to both employers and employees to pay health insurance premiums, and to employers for provider claims paid in self-insured plans. The total cost to the US Federal government for providing the employer-sponsored health insurance exclusion was about $273 billion in 2019.

FIGURE 01.1: VISUAL CHAPTER SUMMARY

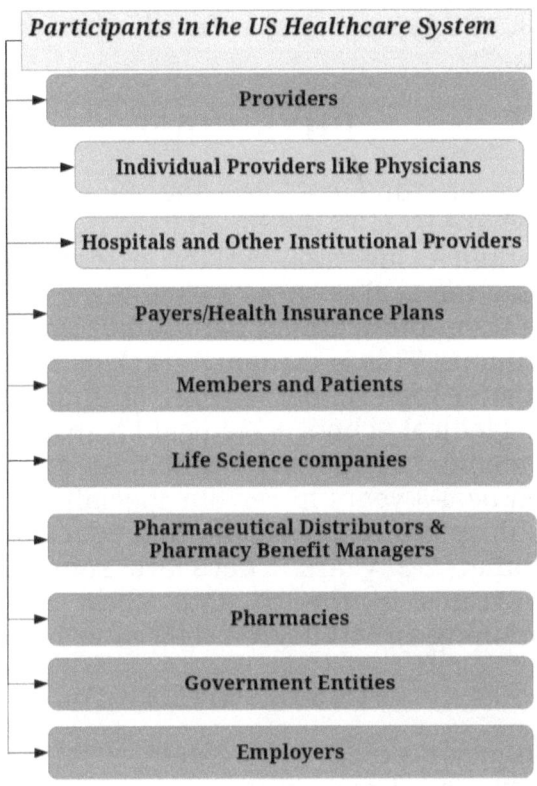

2. INDIVIDUAL PROVIDERS

There are many types of individual providers in healthcare but we will look at 3 types in more detail: physicians, nurses, and pharmacists.

PHYSICIANS

Physicians or "doctors" are the face of the healthcare system. They are usually the healthcare professionals with the greatest amount of decision-making power when it comes to detailing what medical services a person should receive.

The education and training path to becoming a physician is long and arduous. This is the usual track in the US to becoming a physician after high school: 4 years of undergraduate college + 4 years of Medical School + Medical Licensing Examination + 3 years of medical residency. Residencies are usually 3 years long but can be 4-5 years in certain specialties. If one wants to become a sub-specialist physician, that requires a fellowship – usually another 2-3 years. There are some 6-8 year Direct Medical programs in the US that allow students to work towards obtaining an MD degree right after high school.[10]

Types of Physicians

The residency decides, to an extent, what kind of physician one becomes. There are various specialties for physicians – internal medicine, pediatrics, dermatology, family practice, emergency medicine, ophthalmology, general surgery, etc. After residency, a fellowship is required to become a sub-specialist. As an example, a cardiologist is usually someone who has completed a fellowship in cardiology after finishing a residency in internal medicine.

Quirks related to physician compensation

Physician salary ranges for various specialties and subspecialties are available by geographical region on many websites like Salary.com. However, one aspect of physician compensation may come as a surprise to people in other occupations. In the US, a physician working in a geographically remote area is likely to earn significantly more for the same specialty or sub-specialty than one employed in an urban center. Also, physicians working in *teaching hospitals* are likely to earn less than their counterparts in private or community hospitals. Lastly, employed physicians are likely to earn significantly less than independent physicians or those in group practices. The trade-off for the physician in the teaching hospital is fewer working hours and less on-call hours (since that is usually handled by residents and fellows) in exchange for lower pay. But the differences can be extreme. One example I often cite is that of a cardiologist who was making $250,000/year in a teaching hospital in Connecticut and moved to a private hospital in Baton Rouge, Louisiana for a compensation package of $750,000/year. Also, employed physicians (who are employees of a hospital or health system) usually make less than physicians having their own practices. This is because physicians with their own practices can bill health insurance companies directly for the services provided to patients (medical billing is discussed in chapter 8). However, the number of independent physician practices has been decreasing in recent years. In the example given above of the cardiologist, an independent (not employed by the institution) interventional cardiologist or electrophysiologist might be able to bill for revenue of $1-$3 million in a year.

One would never expect a computer programmer in the San Francisco Bay area to be making less than one in rural Kansas – but that is exactly what could be the case for physicians!

Primary care in rural areas and small towns, where Medicare and Medicaid are the predominant payers, is the one sector where physician compensation is likely to be much lower than in larger cities. This is because Medicare and Medicaid pay significantly less than private health plans for primary care services.

Another quirk of physician compensation in the US is that years of experience do not count much in deciding how much a physician earns. This is because reimbursement to providers is done by third party payers, and a health insurance plan will pay the same amount for a service or procedure whether it is done by a newbie physician fresh out of their residency, or by a 35-year veteran doctor. Thus, most physicians earn almost the same amounts over their careers. In fact, younger physicians might put in more hours and cover more shifts, and thus be able to earn more than older physicians who are winding down their workloads.

NURSES AND NURSE PRACTITIONERS

Nurses help in the care of patients for bettering or maintaining their health statuses. Nurses perform many functions in healthcare but the three main categories of activities they perform are (i) Assisting patients in the activities of daily living, (ii) Medication administration and carrying out other orders written by physicians, and (iii) Patient education.

There are three major paths to becoming a nurse after high school. The Registered Nurse licensure can be obtained after (i) a two year Associate Degree in Nursing, (ii) a three year diploma, or (iii) a four year Bachelor of Science in Nursing college degree.

Nurses play a critical role in the delivery of healthcare. In most cases, at least in hospital in-patient settings, individuals will have the most interaction with nursing staff among all the healthcare professionals engaged in their care.

Nurse practitioners are mid-level practitioners who are advanced practice registered nurses. Nurse practitioners, in some states, have almost all the practice rights and privileges as physicians. But, in other states they have reduced privileges and have to work under the supervision of a physician.[11]

PHARMACISTS

Pharmacists are healthcare professionals who are trained in the effective use of medications. This includes aspects like medication safety, efficacy, patient education, and drug interactions. Pharmacists can be retail pharmacists (usually dispensing drugs in outpatient pharmacies) or hospital pharmacists. The prerequisite to licensure for a pharmacist involves obtaining a Pharm.D. (Doctor of Pharmacy) degree. Post high-school, this involves 2-4 years of undergraduate college followed by 4 years of the Pharm.D. degree.

PERSON-TO-PERSON SERVICE DELIVERY

One of the unique characteristics of the healthcare system is that, except in some rare cases, the delivery of the medical service or product is person-to-person. This interaction could be physician-to-patient, nurse-to-patient, pharmacist-to-patient, etc. This fact is also one of the reasons that healthcare has not had the levels of automation seen in other industries like retail, finance, and manufacturing. We are still, for example, at least a few years away from having the physician replaced by a computer or a robot.

FIGURE 02.1: VISUAL CHAPTER SUMMARY

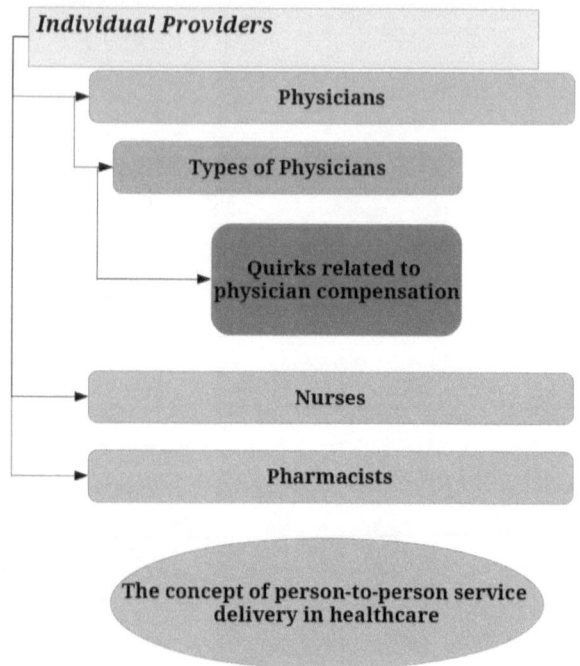

3. HOW A PHYSICIAN WORKS

This chapter aims to provide a simplification of how a physician carries out the clinical processes in his/her purview as part of the healthcare workflow. Even though there are various other healthcare workers involved in the processes that comprise healthcare delivery, I concentrate on the physician because, in the large amount of cases, they take *responsibility* for the care being delivered to a patient: the buck stops with the doctor!

Years of training in medical school, residencies, and fellowships coupled with clinical experience turns physicians into sophisticated pattern-matching experts. But there is still a process ingrained into physicians' clinical workflow that optimizes their time and the results.

The first thing a physician does when he/she sees a new patient is to obtain a detailed **history** of the illness from the patient or the accompanying caregiver/relative. The history starts with what is known as the "chief complaint" or "reason for current visit" and elaborates out everything that the patient describes in terms of symptoms, onset of illness, severity, duration, and other characteristics. All the while the history is being understood by the physician, her brain is engaged in a sophisticated pattern-matching exercise against all the knowledge gained from training and experience – this helps to narrow down the number of areas to focus on and helps in the process of assigning a diagnosis.

The next step is that of **examination** where a physician uses her hands, tools like stethoscopes and otoscopes, and her senses to physically examine the patient. This is done to identify clinical findings that further narrow down the possible-diagnoses down to a few.

Based on the history and examination, a physician will usually have arrived at a **working diagnosis** and a **differential diagnosis.** The differential diagnosis refers to a list of potential diagnoses (clinical conditions) that could all present with the set of history and physical findings that the physician just noted. The working diagnosis is the first diagnosis in the differential diagnosis list. It is the diagnosis that is considered most likely to be the case by the physician and it will drive most of the provisional treatment and diagnostic testing. As an example, a physician might have a working diagnosis of depression for a patient with a differential diagnosis list that includes central nervous system disorders, infectious disease, endocrine disorders, and drug-related conditions.[12]

The physician will then write **orders** down for what needs to be done next. One set of orders will address the provisional treatment – the medications, procedures, and other treatments that will start the curative process for the patient (assuming that the working diagnosis is the correct one). The other set of orders addresses the diagnostic and exploratory tests and examinations that are meant to confirm the working diagnosis and exclude with certainty the items on the differential diagnosis list. These tests include laboratory tests, blood-work and other body fluid examinations, radiological tests, biopsies, genetic tests, and a battery of other potential diagnostic modalities. In many cases, no provisional treatment beyond symptomatic relief is started without diagnostic and exploratory tests. Based on the results of the diagnostic tests, the diagnosis might be revised – in which case the treatment orders for the patient will change. This diagnosis-tests-treatment process might take a few iterations if the patient's condition does not reveal itself to the physician early.

The **diagnosis** is the physician's assessment of the clinical condition that the patient has. **Procedures** are courses of action to be taken for patients as part of their care. These can be *curative/treatment procedures* like surgery, vaccination and dialysis or *diagnostic procedures* like electrocardiography, lab testing, endoscopy, and radiological imaging.

Orders are the method by which the physician outlines the things to be done for the patient. Physician orders include a whole host of things including medication prescriptions, orders for inpatient-administration of drugs, diagnostic and lab tests, consults with other physicians, biopsies, and dietary restrictions. The care team supporting the physician (nurses, pharmacists, physician assistants, lab technicians and others) help in the execution of many of the orders. The patient is also responsible for carrying out many of the ordered items – especially when the patient sees the physician in a clinic setting and then goes back home.

The other big item on the physician's to-do list is **clinical documentation**. All of the clinical processes carried out for the patient, starting with the history and physical, have to recorded by the physician and other clinical staff as clinical documentation. There are several standard clinical notes for this purpose – like "History and Physical", "Admission Note", "Emergency Room Note", "Discharge Summary", "Progress Note", etc. For a lot of the notes, the physicians and other clinical staff use the **SOAP** note methodology. **SOAP** is an acronym for Subjective-Objective-Assessment-Plan. The *subjective* part of the SOAP note consists of the chief complaint, the history of illness, social history, family history, and other information that the physician gathers through the interview. The *objective* part of the SOAP note consists of the information related to vital signs (blood pressure, body temperature, pulse, respiratory rate, height, weight), physical examination findings, medication history, and already-available results from previous lab and diagnostic tests. The *assessment* includes the working diagnosis and the differential diagnosis list previously described as well as the physician's evaluation of risk factors, progress so far, treatment issues, etc. The *plan* describes what the physician recommends as further treatment and tests for the patient.

HEALTHCARE DELIVERY LOCATIONS

Healthcare delivery locations or settings can broadly be categorized into two types: **Outpatient** and **Inpatient**.

Outpatient Setting

Outpatient healthcare settings include all the locations where a patient is considered as ***not admitted*** into a healthcare facility. This usually means that the patient is not occupying a bed in the hospital or healthcare facility. However, there are cases where the patient might be in a bed but still considered an outpatient e.g. when receiving **Observation Services** in a hospital to gauge whether admission is necessary. Examples of outpatient settings include:
1. Physician Clinic
2. Emergency Department also known as an Emergency Room
3. Observation services in a hospital
4. Outpatient surgery center
5. Lab testing facility
6. Radiological Imaging Facility

Inpatient Setting

Inpatient healthcare settings include situations where the patient is **admitted** to a hospital with a physician's order.

Understanding inpatient and outpatient settings is important because the healthcare-setting controls processes like clinical workflow, billing, and the type of medical claim. These are all things we will discuss later.

INDEPENDENT AND EMPLOYED PHYSICIANS

Independent physicians are those who practice alone or as part of group-practices (group of physicians who form a business entity) as autonomous entities. These physicians have to function like independent businesses and manage their offices themselves. Independent physicians usually acquire **"practice privileges"** for nearby hospitals and other clinical facilities in order to be able to deliver care at these locations. For example, an independent group of critical care physicians might have practice privileges for a particular hospital in the area. This allows the physicians in the group to practice in the intensive care unit of the hospital even though they are not employees of the hospital. The billing for these situations is complicated and explained later in this book.

Employed physicians are salaried employees of a hospital or health system. They are not independent business entities. Thus, they do not have to manage tasks like running their offices and billing for their professional services. Their employer (the hospital or health system) manages these tasks for them.

Employed physicians usually make less in terms of compensation than independent physicians – the trade-off being that they do not have to deal with the headache of running a business. A lot of previously independent physicians have closed their practices and joined health systems as employees. This is part of a growing trend. The percentage of independent physicians decreased from 57% in 2000 to about 33% at the end of 2016.[13]

FIGURE 03.1: VISUAL CHAPTER SUMMARY

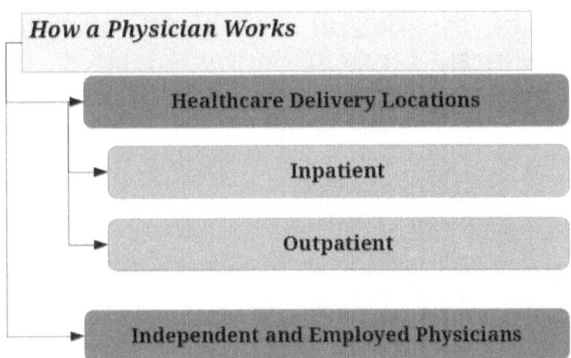

4. CLINICAL DATA

Clinical data can be defined as data generated as a *direct* consequence of the delivery of healthcare. Therefore, the physician **orders**, **clinical notes**, lab-test **results**, and medication **prescriptions** discussed previously are all clinical data subject-areas. On the other hand, medical claims (which we will discuss later) are not considered to be clinical data since they are generated as part of a secondary activity (medical billing/reimbursement and revenue cycle operations) and are not *directly* related to the provision of healthcare. There are some types of data, like pharmacy claims, which are in a gray area: these can be considered both clinical and claims data. This is because pharmacy claims are generated as a direct consequence of the provision of healthcare (dispensing of the prescription) even though they support a healthcare reimbursement process.

There are various subject areas of clinical data.

1. Allergies: A patient's allergies refer to the substances (including drugs, food items, and other allergens) that the individual might have adverse reactions and sensitivities to.
2. Problems: Clinical conditions that a physician wants to track for a patient. Problems usually are the conditions that stay with the patient and are not associated with just a single clinical encounter.
3. Procedures: Surgical, interventional, diagnostic, or therapeutic actions carried out for the patient.
4. Diagnoses: The clinical conditions pertinent to a clinical encounter.
5. Family history: Clinical history of the family of the patient.
6. Social history: Social and cultural information about the patient which might guide diagnosis and treatment.
7. Payer information: Information about the patient's health insurance policy or health plan coverage.
8. Advance directives: Contain the patient's instructions on how to proceed in case he/she is no longer able to make decisions for himself/herself because of illness or incapacitation.
9. Medications: Drugs and similar pharmaceutical agents prescribed or administered to the patient.

10. Immunizations: Vaccines and similar pharmaceutical agents administered to the patient.
11. Medical equipment: The patient's internal and external medical devices and equipment.
12. Vital signs: The patient's objective readings relating to blood pressure, heart rate, respiratory rate, height, weight, body mass index, head circumference, crown-to-rump length, and pulse oximetry. Some of these are only applicable to children.
13. Functional status: The patient's state of functioning. Includes information about mental status, mobility and ambulation, activities of daily living, and home-support status.
14. Results (Lab and other): Information from laboratory and other tests being carried out on the patient.
15. Encounters: An encounter (clinical encounter) is an instance of a patient's interaction with a healthcare provider. It usually occurs in a healthcare setting like a clinic or a hospital. An encounter can be short (clinic office visit) or last many months/years (like a long inpatient hospitalization or confinement).
16. Appointments: Scheduled calendar-dates for planned clinical encounters. A scheduled appointment may or may not result in an encounter.
17. Orders: The instructions relating to the things to be done for the patient.
18. Clinical Notes/Documents: Clinical documentation that outlines the patient's condition and records details of the healthcare services delivered.
19. Plan of care: Details out future orders, interventions, procedures and the like for the patient.

Though the original purpose of the document was different, the HITSP C154 online resource provides a good introduction to the fields that make up the various clinical data subject[14] areas.

Compared to payer data, which we will read about in chapter 9, clinical data is *rich* but not *wide*. This means that for individual patients and health-system encounters, clinical data describes in full detail what transpired during the course of the encounter. However, clinical data is usually limited to a particular health system or provider, while a patient can visit many different providers during the course of seeking healthcare services. Thus, unless a Health Information

Exchange or similar entity is aggregating the data from multiple providers, clinical data will usually not provide a comprehensive account of the healthcare received by a patient/member. Payer data (comprised mostly of medical and pharmacy claims received by payers from providers), which is described in chapter 9, is more *wide* than *rich:* because all the providers that a patient/member sees submit reimbursement claims to the same payer. However, provider claims are not as detailed in the information they contain compared to clinical data.

In the next chapter, we will read about the primary place where clinical data is stored: the patient chart. We will also learn about the digital representation of the patient chart as Electronic Medical Records (EMRs).

FIGURE 04.1: VISUAL CHAPTER SUMMARY

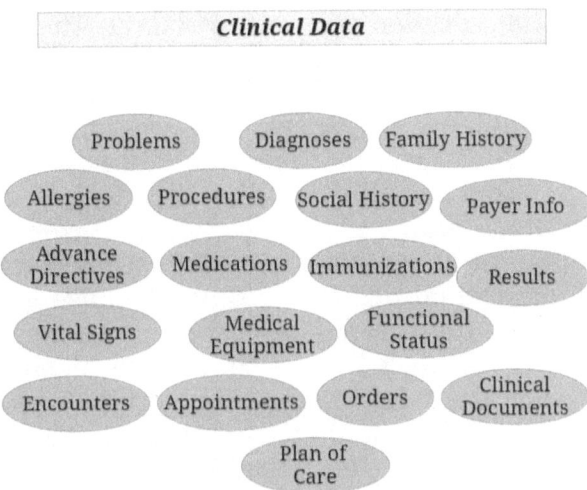

5. THE PATIENT CHART AND EMRs

Clinical information about a patient is stored at a particular provider in what is called the **patient chart**. The patient chart has information on all the patient's visits to the provider, and other clinical data of the kind discussed earlier in the book: medications, problems, diagnoses, allergies, etc.

The patient chart used to be maintained in paper form at a particular provider location. While this was a manageable arrangement for the physician or provider, it came with many issues. The patient chart could only be accessed, managed, or updated by a single clinician at a time. Because large parts of the chart were handwritten, it was sometimes illegible. Charts could get lost or displaced since they were in physical paper form. Because of these and many other problems with the use of paper charts, digital methods to store patient information started being developed a few decades back. Electronic Medical Records or EMRs are digital representations of the patient chart. The phrase Electronic Health Record (EHR) is used interchangeably with the phrase Electronic Medical Record. However, here is a slight difference between an EMR and an EHR: the EMR represents the digital patient chart at a provider while the EHR represents the total health information of the patient. Another way to describe this is to say that an EHR is an EMR that allows sharing and use (interoperability) of the digital patient information across multiple providers and the patient herself. Over the past few decades, EMR/EHR adoption has increased tremendously. As of 2015, about 87% of US office-based physicians were using EHRs.[15]

Also, as of 2015 again, 96% of US non-federal acute care hospitals were using certified EHRs.[16]

Many different vendors make EHR systems. Some of the popular ones include Cerner, Epic, Meditech, AllScripts, NextGen, eClinicalworks, and PracticeFusion. The Veterans Affairs branch of the Federal Government has a home-grown EHR system named VistA.

ADVANTAGES OF EMRs/EHRs

EHR systems offer several advantages over patient charts.
1. Since the patient clinical information is stored in digital form, EMR systems address the issues relating to

storage, loss, and displacement of paper patient charts. Obviously however, a Health Information Technology (IT) infrastructure is required to support an EHR system.

2. A single patient's EHR chart can be accessed, managed, and updated simultaneously by multiple physicians and other healthcare workers engaged in caring for the patient. This is because the physical limitation of having to send the patient chart around is bypassed.
3. Problems with legibility are addressed: most of the information is typed in.
4. Patient safety is improved through a decrease in medical errors. One reason is legibility and the ability for the electronic patient chart to be simultaneously read by multiple clinicians – many eyes on the same information leads to a decrease in errors. Also, sophisticated EHR systems have clinical decision support alerts programmed into them for addressing medication errors, allergy alerts, and many other patient-safety issues.
5. EHRs allow medical billing to proceed faster and with better detail.
6. The digital information stored in the EHR allows analytics and research to be executed at both the patient and population levels.

PROBLEMS OF EMRs/EHRs

All is not rosy in the EHR world though. Many physicians have found it hard to transition from paper charts to digital EHR systems. Several problems have been voiced about EHRs.

1. EHRs are criticized for furthering a cookie-cutter style of practicing medicine where templatized processes and documentation take precedence over the patient-physician interaction.
2. The administrative burden of electronic documentation has increased for physicians because of EHR use.
3. Huge financial investments in health information technology are required to implement and maintain EHR systems.
4. Due to constraints of time and the demands of electronic documentation, physicians find that clinical interaction with patients suffers in both qualitative and

quantitative terms when EHRs are used.
5. The goal of the healthcare Triple Aim[17] (improving the patient experience, improving the health of populations, and decreasing the cost of healthcare), promised through widespread EHR adoption, has not really been achieved.
6. EMR systems are blamed as one of the major reasons for "physician burnout" occurring across the US, since physicians bear the additional, stress-generating, administrative burden of clinical documentation and order entry.

In spite of these issues, EHR systems have had a beneficial effect on healthcare. Therefore, we are unlikely to see a return to paper charts.

CLINICAL STANDARDS IN HEALTH IT

The term *clinical standards*, when applied to Health IT, refers to two different categories of concepts. The first of them covers the representation of clinical data using refined data models, data dictionaries and terminologies, and relationship diagrams. The second category addresses the messaging specifications for the exchange and interoperability of clinical information between organizations, EMR systems, and other clinical and non-clinical systems.

Clinical Data Representation Standards

These standards deal with the data models and the semantic representation of clinical data. An example is the **HL7 version 3 Reference Information Model**. Also included are clinical vocabularies and terminologies used to represent and codify clinical elements. Examples of clinical vocabularies include:
  ➤ SNOMED-CT to represent almost everything in clinical medicine: orders, diagnoses, clinical findings, vital signs, allergies, etc.
  ➤ LOINC for lab results, vital signs, and clinical documents
  ➤ CPT for medical procedures and services
  ➤ ICD9 and ICD10 for diagnoses and facility procedures
  ➤ RxNorm for medications
  ➤ NDC for medications
  ➤ ... *and many more*

Clinical Data Interoperability Standards

These standards help in the exchange, interchange, sharing and interoperability of clinical data between entities like providers, labs, facilities, public health agencies, etc. Examples of these standards include:

- ➢ HL7 version 2 messaging specifications
- ➢ HL7 version 3 messaging specifications
- ➢ FHIR
- ➢ *... and many more*

HL7

The organization HL7[18] has probably done the most in terms of creating, maintaining, and advocating for clinical standards. The HL7 version 2 specifications for the transfer of healthcare information are still the most widely used healthcare messaging standards. HL7 version 3, which came out in 2005, specified standards for not just the transfer but also the representation and semantics of clinical data. Unfortunately, since most EHR systems had created their clinical models much before the HL7 Reference Information Model for clinical data representation was available, there is still a widespread interoperability problem in healthcare when it comes to EHRs. The same clinical data is represented and stored in different ways in EHR systems from diverse vendors. The FHIR standard is a new HL7 standard that seeks to simplify the exchange of clinical data.

FIGURE 05.1: VISUAL CHAPTER SUMMARY

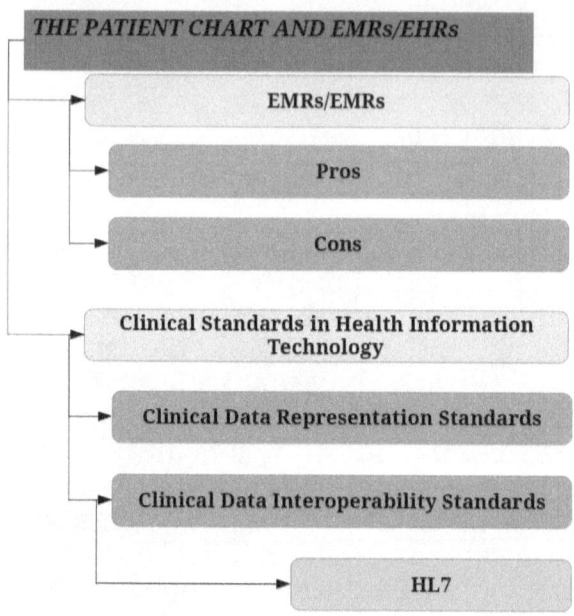

6. HEALTHCARE PAYERS

As outlined in chapter 1, a healthcare payer is usually a private health insurance company/health plan or a government entity. Regardless of this difference, a *payer* pays the *providers* who deliver healthcare services to the *members* covered under the payer's plan. Therefore a *member* is a person who is covered by a payer's health insurance plan. About 9% of the US population is still uninsured,[19] i.e., not covered by any health insurance policy.

A private healthcare payer's revenue comes mostly from *premiums*, the money collected from members on an annual basis to provide *coverage* for the year. In this regard, healthcare insurance works similar to home insurance, or vehicle and other casualty insurance in that premiums are collected from the members/insured. However, the big difference in the US is that vehicle and home insurance are usually catastrophic policies that pay out only in the event of catastrophic damage to an automobile or property. But health insurance policies usually pay for *all* medical care and not just catastrophic care. For example, a vehicle insurance policy will not pay for regular maintenance like oil changes or even major repairs to a car like an alternator change. Similarly, a home insurance policy will not pay for the home to be painted or the driveway re-done. But a health insurance policy is usually expected to cover all healthcare services: preventive as well as catastrophic. Think of a health insurance policy as an extended warranty on a vehicle that covers catastrophic repairs *as well as* oil changes!

Based on the customers that a health insurance company seeks and serves, we can define the concept of the types of *health insurance customer/purchaser markets*. A health insurance consumer market targets specific types of *customers* or *purchasers to sell health insurance plans to*. The three main health insurance markets in the US are Employer, Individual, and Government.

Is Insurance Socialism?

This is an interesting and controversial debate. In one provocative sense, health-insurance (and all other sorts of insurance) can be considered a form of socialism – since the premiums from all the insurance-consumers are pooled but the most money goes towards the care provided to the sickest and the neediest. But, an opposing viewpoint is that health insurance is the best possible free-market solution for managing the clinical and financial risk of a population.

HEALTH INSURANCE CUSTOMER/PURCHASER MARKET TYPES

1. Employer Market

The employer market consists of companies and organizations that want to purchase and provide health insurance coverage to their employees. More than 50% of Americans with health insurance (about 49% of the total US population) get it from their employers. The US tax code provides tax benefits to employers for providing health insurance coverage for their employees. Thus, many employers find it advantageous to offer health insurance benefits to their workers. There are two main types of models in the employer-sponsored health insurance market: fully insured and self insured (self-insured is also sometimes known as ASO: Administrative Services Only).

Fully Insured Employer Health Plans

These are health insurance coverage plans purchased by the employer where the health insurance company is required to pay the provider claims associated with the provision of healthcare. In other words, the financial risk associated with the cost of medical care is assumed by the health insurance company. Thus, in this sort of arrangement, the health insurance company provides the network of providers to deliver care, offers administrative services for the processing of claims and other operations, and assumes the financial risk for the cost of medical care delivered.

Self Insured Employer Health Plans

These are health insurance coverage plans purchased by the employer where the financial risk for the claims associated with the provision of medical care are assumed by the employer rather than the health insurance company. In this arrangement, the health insurance company provides the network of providers and administrative services like claims processing but does not assume the financial risk of medical care claim payment. In some cases, there is a separate "Third Party Administrator" (TPA) which performs the claims processing and other administrative functions for the employer or for the health insurance company that the employer has bought the self-funded plan from.

Small Group, Large Group, and National Accounts

Health insurance companies will usually divide employers' health policies based on the number of employees insured. A small group policy usually covers up to 50 (sometimes 100) employees. A large group policy covers employers with 51 or more employees. And a National Account is a policy for an employer that covers more than 3000 employees.

2. Individual Market

The individual market consists of people who purchase and receive health insurance on their own, and not through an employer or the US Federal or State governments. This constitutes about 6% of the total US population. Before 2010 and the passage of the Affordable Care Act (ACA), people with pre-existing medical conditions found it very difficult to get health insurance coverage in the individual market – health insurance companies would refuse to sell them a policy because of one or more pre-existing medical conditions they had. This process is called medical underwriting. As part of the Affordable Care Act of 2010, medical underwriting was made illegal and *guaranteed issue* of a health insurance policy was ensured.

3. Government Market

The government market consists of people in the US who receive health insurance coverage through a governmental health insurance plan. Several types of governmental health insurance exist and about 35% of the US population gets its health insurance coverage from a governmental plan.

Medicare

Medicare is a US Federal governmental health insurance program that provides coverage to seniors above the age of 65, and some specific groups of individuals like those with End Stage Renal Disease or total and permanent disabilities.

Medicaid

Medicaid is health insurance provided by the US Federal and State governments to poor people. Medicaid is funded by both the Federal government and the state governments.

Military Health Coverage

Health coverage is provided to active duty military personnel and veterans through the Department of Defense's Military Health System and the Veterans Health Administration.

Children's Health Insurance Program (CHIP)

Similar to Medicaid, this is a joint US Federal + state program that provides health coverage to children of low-income families that still have incomes in excess of the threshold below which they qualify for Medicaid.

Indian Health Service

Provides health insurance coverage to Native Americans.

Figure 06.1: Health Insurance Markets

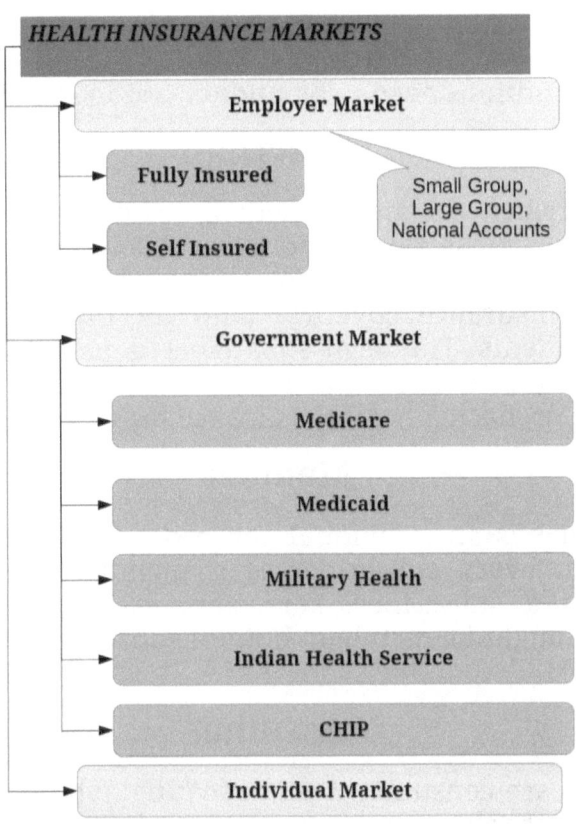

SUBSCRIBERS, MEMBERS, CONSUMERS, AND PATIENTS

Some definitions need to be understood in order to proceed.

Subscriber

A subscriber is an individual who purchases health insurance or whose employment or other arrangement makes them eligible for health insurance coverage. Subscribers might get health insurance coverage both for themselves and for their dependents. The term subscriber is usually used for an individual person though, in rare cases, it might refer to the employer purchasing health insurance for its employees.

Member

A member is an individual covered by a health insurance plan. Thus, every subscriber is a member. But not every member is a subscriber. For example, dependents of the subscriber might be members but not subscribers of the health plan.

Consumer

A healthcare consumer is an individual who is in a position to consume healthcare services (though they might not be doing so at a particular time).

Patient

A patient is a consumer who is actively consuming and/or receiving healthcare services. Thus, all patients are consumers, but not all consumers are patients at a particular point in time.

COSTS FOR HEALTH PLAN MEMBERS

Health plan members (usually the subscribers) bear various costs when they are covered by a health plan.

Premium

This is the fixed monthly amount paid to maintain coverage.

This is similar to a subscription paid to ensure that the health plan covers medical service costs for the member when they arise. In employer-provided health insurance coverage in the US, between 60 to 80 percent of the premium is paid by the employer (which is able to get tax deductions from the US government for this contribution to employee-coverage premiums) and the rest is paid by the employees themselves.

Deductible

This is a monetary amount that the health plan expects the member/subscriber to pay out of pocket before it starts covering the cost of medical services utilized by the member. This deductible does not apply to the costs of preventive care, which are paid from the first dollar onward by the health plan. As an example, a health plan sold in the individual market might have an annual premium of $7,000 and an annual deductible of $4,000 dollars. This means that, excluding preventive care, the member has to pay $11,000 dollars out of pocket for the year before the health plan starts paying for services and care.

Co-Pay

This is a flat monetary amount that is paid every time a member receives care. For example, there might be a $25 co-pay for every physician-office visit by a member. Co-pays usually do not count towards the deductible.

Co-Insurance

This is a percentage amount that is charged from the member for various types of care in different facilities. For example, a health plan might have a 20% co-insurance for emergency-room care – which means that it will only cover 80% of the cost of an emergency room visit. The other 20% will have to be paid by the member. Co-insurance only comes into play after the deductible has been met for the year. Before the deductible is met for the year, the whole cost of such an emergency-room visit will be borne by the member.

Other Costs (like balance billed amounts)

Health insurance plans usually work with the concept of a *provider network*, a list of hospitals, physicians, and other healthcare providers in a geographical area who have agreed to accept discounted payment rates for the care delivered to the members covered by the health plan. In some types of health plans, the seeking of out-of-network care by members is strictly discouraged. However, this can lead to ugly financial situations in which a member is billed by an out-of-network provider for huge sums of money that are not covered by the health plan. It becomes an even more unfair situation when the care is sought in an acute situation like going to an emergency room for a medical emergency. In such situations, the member does not have the liberty or time to make an informed and considered choice. Balance billing has been a hot topic of discussion for consumer advocates. The US government has been looking at laws and rules to prevent balance billing.

Out-of-Pocket-Maximum

This is a monetary cap on the amount that the member will need to pay out-of-pocket if they run up large medical costs. This amount does not include the annual premium but includes the deductible, co-pays, and co-insurance. For example, an individual health policy might have an annual premium of $7,000, an annual deductible of $4,000, and an annual out-of-pocket-maximum of $8,000. This means that if, for some reason, a member incurs large medical services costs, after paying the $7,000 annual premium, and another $8,000 (in deductibles, co-pays, and co-insurance), they will pay no more for the year no matter how high the medical services costs go.

Yearly and Lifetime Payout Limits

These yearly and lifetime payout limits on medical claims were previously enforced by health plans. However, the Affordable Care Act of 2010 stops health insurance companies from enforcing yearly and lifetime payout limits. Thus, they are on the hook for the full extent of a member's healthcare claims.

HEALTHCARE PLANS AND SYSTEMS

There are various types of health plans available along with the health systems that are tied with them. They offer varying degrees of freedom to the member to see any healthcare provider of their choice.

1. Traditional Indemnity Health Insurance Plan (Fee-for-Service or FFS type)

These are the first types of health insurance plans that were available, before plans with restricted provider-networks became popular. The provider network (a term explained later in this book) is the list of healthcare providers that a member can choose from when needing care. In a traditional indemnity health plan, there is no concept of a restricted healthcare provider network. A member can choose whichever provider (hospital, physician, clinic, etc..) they like. The health insurance company pays what are known as *usual/reasonable and customary* charges for every healthcare service. If this is less than what the provider bills for, the balance is paid by the member. Such plans, as you can imagine, leave the member/patient on the hook for potential differences between the usual and customary rate and what the provider might bill. Traditional indemnity health plans are extremely rare in the US now, because they have been superseded by the network-type plans.

2. Preferred Provider Organization (PPO) type plan

The PPO is the most accommodating of the types of health plans that fall under the *managed care* umbrella. A PPO has a listed network of providers that the plan has contracted with. However, the member can see (visit for clinical services) a provider out of the network although the out-of-pocket costs will be higher than in-network. Also, there is no assigned Primary Care Physician (PCP) for every member, and no referral from a primary care provider is required to see a specialist. The premiums for a PPO plan are higher than for other managed care plans. And seeing out-of-network providers is still costly for members because they might get hit with balance billed amounts and higher deductibles to satisfy.

3. Exclusive Provider Organization (EPO) type plan

The EPO is a managed care plan that is more restrictive than a PPO. The member is only allowed to see providers within the defined network. If the member sees a provider outside of the defined network (except for emergency care), they are responsible for bearing the full cost. A primary care physician is usually assigned to each member. However, a referral from a primary care physician is not usually required for a member to see a specialist. Premiums are lower than with PPO plans but deductibles and co-pays might be higher.

4. Health Maintenance Organization (HMO) type plan

The HMO is the most restrictive of the managed care plans. Members can see providers only within their network. Any out-of-network care costs are completely the member's responsibility, except for emergency care. A primary care physician is assigned to each member and members require referrals from their primary care doctors in order to see specialists in their network. Premiums are the lowest compared to the other managed care type plans. There are four main types of HMO plans.

I. Group Model HMO

A Group Model HMO involves a plan that contracts with a single multiple-specialty group practice of providers. The plan usually pays the medical group a capitated dollar amount (an educated guess based on actuarial calculations of what medical costs for the member population are likely to be in the year) which is distributed to the physicians in the practice group in some sort of salary+incentive formula. In this arrangement, the medical group has to make an effort to hold medical costs for its HMO population within a certain limit. However, the medical group might also be providing care to non-HMO populations of patients/members.

II. Staff Model HMO

A Staff Model HMO is one in which the physicians are employees (staff) of the health plan. The health plan also usually owns the facilities in which medical services are provided.

III. Network Model HMO

A Network Model HMO is a health plan that contracts with multiple medical practice groups to provide services to its members. The medical groups might also be providing care to non-HMO members.

IV. Independent Practice Association (IPA) HMO

An IPA is a business entity formed by the coming together of multiple independent medical practice groups, in order to contract with a managed care organization or health plan. An IPA can be broad and community based or narrower and hospital based. The IPA contracts with the HMO plan to provide services to the HMO members. The IPA might also contract with non-HMO plans and provide services to those members.

4. Point of Service (POS) type plan

The POS is a managed care plan that is a blend of the HMO and the PPO. There is more choice within the network of providers, but primary care physicians are assigned to all members and PCP referrals are required to see specialists. Out of network care can be sought by members but is more costly for them.

5. High Deductible Health Plan (HDHP)

The HDHP involves, as the name indicates, higher deductibles in return for lower premiums. The HDHP plan can be a PPO, EPO, HMO, or POS plan. In many HDHPs, a Health Savings Account (HSA) can be set up that allows contributions of tax-free dollars by the member and their employer to use for paying for medical care later.

6. Catastrophic Plan

A catastrophic plan is only available to individuals under the age of 30 years or those who qualify for a hardship exemption like homelessness, bankruptcy, and eviction. Such a plan mainly covers serious emergency illnesses, accidents, and hospitalizations but has limited coverage of preventive care and primary care.

7. Short Term Health Plan

A short term health plan provides temporary medical care coverage in special situations like when someone is between plans or outside an enrollment period. These provide limited health benefits and will not provide coverage in case of pre-existing conditions. These should be used only in very special situations as they are not long term alternatives to standard health insurance plans.

Figure 06.2: Healthcare Plans and Systems

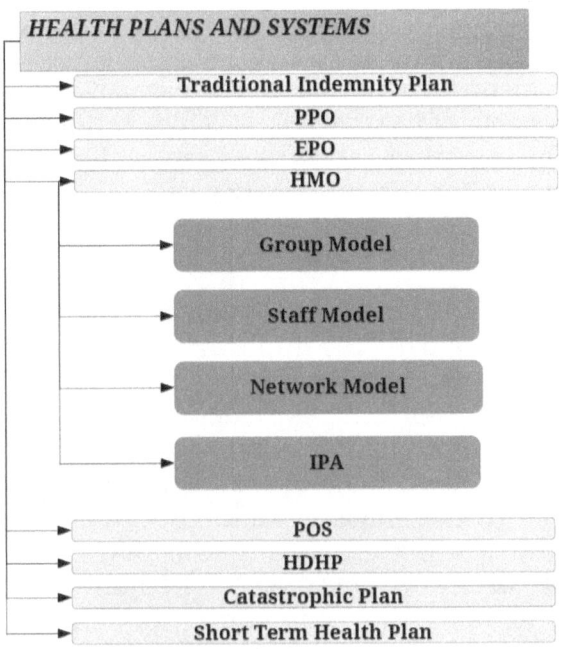

PAYER PROCESSES AND TERMINOLOGY/DEFINITIONS

A health insurance plan (payer) carries out a number of processes as parts of its operations. This section describes some of the major business tasks and activities at payers, and explains some of the common jargon and terms encountered.

1. Underwriting

This refers to the process of evaluating and taking on the financial risk of insuring the applicant or applicant-population. Once the decision to insure an applicant has been made, the amount of the premium is calculated based on further actuarial calculations of risk. Before the Affordable Care Act (ACA) of 2010, health insurers could carry out *medical underwriting,* which means that they could evaluate an applicant's health status, health history, and pre-existing conditions in order to determine whether to issue coverage and what to set the premium to. However, *medical underwriting* has been prohibited by the ACA and so has denial of coverage due to pre-existing conditions. What is used now is underwriting based on *community rating,* where premiums can vary only on the basis of geographical area, age, and tobacco use. Also, there is a ceiling on the ratio between the highest and lowest premium charged for applicants with the same insurance plan. In addition, *guaranteed issue* is now the law of the land for regular health insurance – which means that the issuance of a policy cannot be denied on the basis of pre-existing conditions or other factors. Another practice called *rescission* used to be common in the health insurance world before the ACA: it refers to the practice of canceling an insured policy retroactively and denying a payout if there was anything incorrect or incomplete found on the original application for insurance. Since *rescission,* which was meant to actually protect health insurance companies from fraud, was misused a lot by plans, the ACA made *rescission* illegal in most cases.

Medical underwriting is still used by health policies not covered by the ACA, like short term plans and supplemental insurance plans. Many of these non-ACA policy products allow the plan to also deny coverage based on pre-existing conditions.

2. Eligibility

Eligibility refers to health insurance eligibility. Members sign up for a health plan during the enrollment period (the last 2-3 months of the previous calendar year) or in special enrollment periods (which might be due to job changes, marital status changes, and other reasons). However, the health plan has to keep track of a member's eligibility every day of the year that they are supposed to be covered. Non payment of premiums and other factors can be reasons for loss of health insurance plan eligibility for a member. This is very important, as a non-eligible member's medical services costs will not be paid by the health plan. This is also the reason why providers sometimes check the eligibility of patients/members with the insurance company whose information is given to them. As part of processing provider-claim payments, an eligibility check is one of the first things done by the health plan.

3. Claims Processing

When a member seek and receives medical care from a provider (physician, health system, hospital, etc.), the invoice for at least part of the payment is sent in the form of a health insurance *medical claim* by the provider to the health plan. This claim, which is usually submitted digitally nowadays (though paper submissions are also allowed), has the details of the patient/member, the medical services provided, the dates of the services, the member/patient's diagnoses, and other information. The health plan then processes this *claim* and makes the payment to the provider if it finds everything in order. If the claim documentation is not in order, the plan might deny the claim, ask for more information, or request re-submission. Specialized information technology systems are used by health plans for claims processing. *Pharmacy claims*, for outpatient prescriptions, follow a similar but separate claims processing pipeline.

3. Claims Adjudication

Claim adjudication is one of the most important parts of claim processing by a health insurance plan. When a claim is submitted by a provider, the health plan evaluates and adjudicates the claim in order to decide whether to pay it in full, deny it, or reduce the payment amount. Denial of payment or reduction of the payment amount could be because of multiple reasons including: Member not eligible, Billing service codes and diagnoses codes for the member are inadequate or supplied incorrectly, Health plan suspects fraud, etc.

4. Coordination of Benefits

Coordination of Benefits (COB) is the process used to make healthcare claim payouts when a person is covered under more than one health insurance plan. Examples of this might be when an individual is a dual-eligible, covered under both Medicare and Medicaid, or a child/dependent of parents who both have access to a health insurance plan, etc.

5. Subrogation

Subrogation is the process by which a health insurance company might legally pursue a third party for insurance losses (medical expenses) incurred. An example is if a member is injured in a traffic accident where the other driver is at fault. In this case, the health insurance company will pay the medical expense claims for the treatment of the member, but might legally pursue the at-fault party (or his/her vehicle insurance company) for recovering the medical expenses incurred.

6. Payment Integrity (Fraud and Abuse)

Payment integrity encompasses all the processes that ensure that erroneous, fraudulent, abusive, and wasteful claims are identified and either denied or recovered after payment. This department of a health plan includes sophisticated analytics and data mining/rules engine processes similar to those used by credit card companies to detect and prevent fraud. The primary aim of payment integrity is to identify such fraudulent claims by providers and stop their payment. But, in some cases, it also involves recovering/clawing back already-paid amounts and initiating criminal action against the perpetrators through coordination with law enforcement.

7. Network Management

A provider network is the network of providers (physicians,

hospitals, health systems, clinics, practices, pharmacies, etc.) that are contracted to a particular health plan in order to provide care to its members. Networks are by definition geographically local, since healthcare is usually delivered locally. However, large health insurance companies can have networks in many states and geographical locations. In the health plan context, the providers with whom it has contractual relationships are called "in-network" while those who are not contracted with are "out-of-network". Usually, a provider contracting with a health plan involves an agreement to provide care to its members at discounted rates rather than the regular billed rates of the providers. The function of network management within a health plan seeks to work with the contracted providers to (a) Reduce healthcare costs, (b) Improve clinical quality, and (c) Improve the satisfaction of the members who receive care. As part of network management contracts, providers might be given additional bonuses at the end of the year for holding down medical costs or delivering quality service. In addition, efforts are always made by the health plan to evaluate providers on the basis of quality and efficiency (with regard to medical costs), and favorable contract renewals are made available to providers who are better on these parameters. A network in a geographical region might be made up of multiple provider entities, but the plan contracts with most of them individually. Thus, network contracting is a big task for the health plan and the providers whose participation is being solicited.

8. Utilization Management

Utilization Management or Utilization Review is a set of processes used by health plans to manage healthcare costs by evaluating clinical services before or as they are delivered, using evidence-based medical guidelines. The appropriateness of care being sought is evaluated as part of this process, and denials or approvals are issued. Two main evidence-based guidelines frameworks are in use in the US: Change Healthcare InterQual®, and MCG Care Guidelines. Utilization management staff in a health insurance plan usually include reviewers (who are usually registered nurses), program managers, and physician advisers. Utilization Management can be done in a *prospective, concurrent,* or *retrospective* manner. Some concepts are important in utilization review/management. One is that of *medical necessity.*[20]

Medical Necessity is a requirement a medical service or procedure is deemed to satisfy if it is reasonable, necessary, and/or appropriate. Another is the process of *prior authorization.* This, as the name implies, involves the provider seeking permission/approval to carry out a service or prescribe a medication, to ensure that the health plan will cover it for the member.

9. Care Management (Case Management & Disease Management)

Care Management can be thought of as an umbrella term that includes both case management and disease management (though some might argue that care management is distinct from the other two). Care Management involves care coordination for members of a managed care health plan.

Case Management is a process to manage the delivery of healthcare services for managed care plan members. Case Management identifies and targets high financial and clinical risk members. These members are those who usually have serious medical issues and/or combinations of social determinants of health that make the coordination of care for these individuals challenging.

Disease Management is similar to case management in terms of providing care coordination to manage healthcare service-delivery, but is for members with one major disease/diagnosis – usually a chronic disease like diabetes, coronary artery disease, asthma, Chronic Obstructive Pulmonary Disease, or one of many others.[21]

A case manager or disease manager is usually a registered nurse assigned to coordinate care for a member. Most of the interactions are telephonic. The various set of activities that a case or disease manager might carry out include: Coordinating with out-of-network providers and negotiating rates, referrals to specialists, special services arrangements, claims coordination, and scheduling important tests and screenings.

In all forms of care management, one of the early steps is called *"Identification and Stratification"*. This involves the utilization of data analytics and health-status assessments to *identify* members who need to be enrolled into care management programs, and to *stratify* them into different clinical and financial risk levels based on the amount of healthcare services they are likely to need.

Also, care management involves identifying clinical care gaps/care opportunities for members and making sure that the services that fill those gaps are made available to them.

10. Risk Adjustment

Risk Adjustment is the process of assigning financial risk scores to all members (based on their clinical conditions, age, social factors, etc.) that help predict the monetary amount of medical care a particular member is likely to require compared to an average member. As an example, if the annual average healthcare expenditure per member in a plan is $10,000, a member with a risk score of 1.0 is likely to utilize $10,000 in medical care in a year. But a member with a risk score of 0.75 is likely to utilize $7,500 and a member with a risk score of 1.25 is likely to utilize $12,500 of medical care in a year. Risk Adjustment is specifically done in plans that come under the Affordable Care Act, and also in Medicare Advantage and Medicaid plans. Risk scoring is also done as part of the actuarial analysis of the member population, in order to figure out the financial risk in terms of medical costs that the health plan might have to bear.

Risk Adjustment is a permanent part of the 2010 Affordable Care Act's processes. It seeks to safeguard against individual and small group health plans' *risk-selection* (usually intentional cherry picking of low-cost members by health plans) and *adverse-selection* (usually unintentional selection of high-cost/high-risk members by health plans without knowing of the actual risk profile) effects. In the Affordable Care Act's risk adjustment program, a plan's average actuarial risk is calculated from the risk-profiles of all its members. Payments flow from lower-risk plans to higher-risk plans and net to zero.

11. Reserving

A claims reserve is money kept aside by a health insurance company in order to pay claims for healthcare services delivered to its members. The process of reserving is required by law for health and other insurance companies. In the case of self-insured health plans, where the claims are paid by the employer, the reserving will be done by the employer. Claims can be *Reported But Not Settled* (RBNS) or *Incurred But Not Reported* (IBNR). Calculation of the amounts to reserve require sophisticated estimation procedures like the *chain ladder* method or the *completion factor* method, along with statistical probability analyses.

12. Medical Loss Ratio/Medical Cost Ratio

The Medical Loss Ratio or MLR (also called the Medical Cost Ratio or MCR) is the ratio of total claims paid or reserved plus adjustment costs to the premiums collected. The Affordable Care Act of 2010 imposed a "floor" (minimum) of 80% for small-group and individual market plans and 85% for large group plans. If the floor is not met, the health plan is mandated to issue rebates to consumers.

13. Reinsurance

Reinsurance is a way for health insurance companies to protect themselves from very high monetary-value claims. A health plan will buy reinsurance coverage from a reinsurance company. As an example, this reinsurance might cover all medical claim costs above $250,000 in a year for any particular member. This is a way for the health insurance company to manage the risk of very-high cost claimants.

Reinsurance was a part of the Affordable Care Act's processes from 2014 to 2016. The idea was that if a plan enrollee's medical costs exceeded a certain threshold (the attachment cost), the plan was eligible to receive payments (up to a cap) to cover this situation. Like with the Affordable Care Act's Risk Adjustment program, payments would net to zero among plans.

14. Stop-Loss Insurance

Stop-loss insurance is similar to reinsurance but is usually purchased by self-insured employers to limit their risk-exposure to high-cost medical claims. Stop-loss insurance can be *specific* (for covering high-cost claims above a certain dollar amount for any particular member) or *aggregate* (that gets activated when a particular dollar amount is exceeded in total for the whole insured population of individuals).

14. Risk Corridors

The Risk Corridors program was part of the Affordable Care Act's processes from 2014 to 2016. It covered plans offered on the health insurance exchanges. The idea was to limit losses and gains and have them be bound within a band. The Health and Human Services department of the Federal Government would collect money from health plans with lower-than-expected medical claims costs and make payments to health plans with higher-then-expected claims costs. Payments would net to zero across plans.

15. Insurance Exchanges

Insurance Exchanges are online exchanges that sell health insurance plans. Public exchanges were set up as part of the Affordable Care Act of 2010 to sell individual, family, and small-group policies directly. These public exchanges were state-run in some states while other states' members were served by the Federal Health Insurance Exchange called Healthcare.gov. Small-group policies have not been available on the Federal Government exchange after 2017.

There are also private insurance exchanges that usually serve large employers when they are purchasing health insurance plans for their employees.

16. Lifetime and Yearly Maximum

Lifetime and yearly maximums used to be limits that health insurance companies could impose on medical claims payouts for a member. However, the Affordable Care Act of 2010 eliminated them, and lifetime and yearly maximums can no longer be applied by health plans.

17. Pre-existing Conditions

A pre-existing condition is a chronic disease or other health condition that a member has when applying for a health insurance policy. In the past, health insurance companies could refuse to issue a policy if an individual had specific pre-existing conditions. However, the Affordable Care Act of 2010 makes it illegal for health insurance companies to refuse to issue policies based on pre-existing conditions.

18. Guaranteed Issue

Guaranteed Issue is the situation when a health plan cannot refuse to issue a health insurance policy to an applicant based on health status or pre-existing conditions. The Affordable Care

Act of 2010 enforces guaranteed issue for all health insurance policies sold.

19. Community Rating

Community rating is the rule enforced by the Affordable Care Act of 2010 that ensures that health insurance companies cannot charge higher premiums for certain members based on factors like health status, pre-existing conditions, previous medical claims history, gender, or many other reasons that the plans used to utilize in the past. However, plans can still adjust premiums for individuals based on age, geographical region, family size, and tobacco-use status. Also, the Affordable Care Act enforces another rule: for age differences in the premium, the highest premium charged within a health insurance policy can be no higher than 3 times the lowest premium charged.

20. Coverage or Benefit Mandates

The Affordable Care Act of 2010 ensures that all plans sold in the exchanges cover specific essential benefits like ambulatory care, emergency services, mental health services, hospitalization, etc. This is known as a coverage or benefit mandate that is enforced by the law.

21. Individual Mandate

An individual mandate is one that forces all individuals living in a country to purchase health insurance or pay a tax penalty for not doing so. An individual mandate was imposed as part of the Affordable Care Act of 2010 on all individuals but was repealed by Congress later, and it is no longer active after 1st January, 2019. However, some states have individual mandates of their own and impose tax penalties for not having health insurance.

22. Employer Mandate

The Affordable Care Act of 2010 requires employers with more than 50 employees to offer health insurance coverage to their employees. Failure by the employer to offer health insurance coverage attracts monetary penalties. This is known as the employer mandate.

23. Medicaid Expansion

The Affordable Care Act of 2010 expanded Medicaid coverage for individuals such that low-income persons would qualify for coverage if their incomes were up to 138% of the Federal Poverty Level.[22]

States were free to adopt the Medicaid expansion for their residents and about two-thirds of US states have chosen to do so this far.

24. Premium Subsidies to Help Individuals Buy Insurance

The Affordable Care Act of 2010 offers tax-credits as subsidies to help pay health insurance premiums for individuals making an annual income of 100% to 400% of the Federal Poverty Level. The lower limit is 138% instead of 100% in US states that have adopted the Medicaid Expansion of the Affordable Care Act.

25. Cost-sharing reductions

In addition to premium tax credit subsidies, the Affordable Care Act (ACA) offered cost-sharing reduction subsidies to low-income individuals to help them deal with out-of-pocket expenses like deductibles, co-pays, and co-insurance. These subsidies were available on a specific category of ACA plans known as "Silver" plans (the other categories being "Gold" and "Bronze"). The Federal government cut off funding for cost-sharing reduction subsidies in October 2017 but most health insurance companies dealt with this situation by adding the cost-sharing reduction amounts to the premiums charged of the members.

7. SPECIAL PROVIDER-RELATED ENTITIES AND CONCEPTS

Several special provider entities have been created for improving business processes and profitability at provider organizations and institutions. Many of these are important in the move towards *payer-provider convergence* – which refers to a healthcare market situation where the differentiation between payers and providers is blurred.

PHYSICIAN HOSPITAL ORGANIZATION

A Physician Hospital Organization (PHO) is a legal and business entity created by physician groups and a hospital coming together. This single organization/entity is able to negotiate better contracts with health plans. A PHO might own and operate other entities like health plans as well.

INTEGRATED DELIVERY NETWORK

An integrated delivery network is an entity comprised of providers and facilities that also owns and operates a health plan. As the phenomenon of payer-provider convergence gains ground, after the Affordable Care Act of 2010, we see more providers and health systems willing to enter the realm of starting financial-risk-bearing health insurance plans. However, bearing the financial risk of health insurance is a complicated and sophisticated process, and it will be interesting to see how many of these previously pure-providers will be successful. In addition, we are also witnessing the phenomenon of health insurance companies buying up provider organizations, thereby becoming dual-function entities.

MANAGEMENT SERVICES ORGANIZATION (MSO)

An MSO is an entity that provides services to a provider organization. These services can include practice management, administrative support, care management, financial management, network management, credentialing, compliance, etc. As health plans pass on the financial risk of members on to providers and health systems they contract with (as part of the concept and process of Population Health, which is explained later), MSOs help providers deal with the back-end and non-clinical processes of managing this risk.

PROVIDER NETWORKS AND NARROW-NETWORK PLANS

In order to control healthcare costs, health plans are offering what are known as "narrow-network plans". As the name indicates, these offer a limited choice of low-cost providers in the geographical area in return for lower premium payments for the members. A narrow-network health plan might include only 10-25% of the providers in a given area, versus the usual approximately 70% offered by traditional health plans. Also, a narrow network plan might have **no** coverage available for out-of-network providers, which leaves members on the hook for the whole billed amount if they decide to see providers who are not part of the health plan's network.

TRIPLE AIM

The Triple Aim[17] is an aspirational goal for healthcare in the US, first proposed by the Institute for Healthcare Improvement. The three parts of the triple aim are: (1) Patient Experience (quality and satisfaction); (2) Improving the health of populations; (3) Reducing the per-person cost of healthcare.

Figure 07.1: The Healthcare Triple Aim

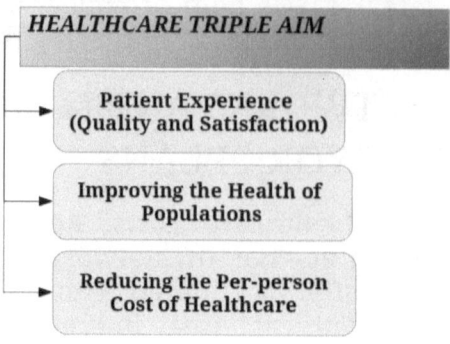

POPULATION HEALTH & ACCOUNTABLE CARE ORGANIZATIONS

According to Kindig and Stoddart (2003), population health is "the health outcomes of a group of individuals, including the distribution of such outcomes within the group". In other words, population health is a process to achieve the previously discussed "Triple Aim" of Healthcare. Accountable Care Organizations (ACOs) are healthcare entities where the reimbursements to providers are linked to both healthcare quality metrics and reductions achieved in the costs of care. Thus, in another sense, ACOs are trials of the 'Value Based Reimbursement' model for providers, where holding down medical costs becomes part of the providers' goal. Thus, an ACO is a set of providers (physicians, hospitals, practice groups, labs, etc.) that contract with a health plan to have their reimbursement tied both to quality as well as holding down medical costs. The ACO model is in contrast to the traditional fee-for-service model, where a provider is reimbursed by the health plan for all rendered services and procedures. *Value Based Reimbursement* is explained further later in this book.

8. MEDICAL BILLING AND PAYMENT

The Medical Billing process followed by providers and its interaction with the reciprocal claim payment/reimbursement process carried out by payers is one of the most complicated parts of the US healthcare system. According to Kevin Quinn writing in the Annals of Internal Medicine (Vol. 163 No. 4, 18 August 2015), there are 8 main methods of healthcare payment in the US.[23]

These 8 payment methods are: (1) Per time period, (2) Per beneficiary, (3) Per recipient, (4) Per episode, (5) Per day, (6) Per service, (7) Per dollar of cost, and (8) Per dollar of charges. Of these, types 4-8 together can be called *Fee for Service* (FFS) Payment and it is the most common method of payment in the US.

FEE FOR SERVICE BILLING AND PAYMENT

Fee for Service (FFS) billing and payment is a model in which each individual service or procedure performed by a provider for a member/patient is reimbursed by the health payer. Out of the payment methods 4-8 above that can be categorized under FFS, the archetype of FFS is type 6: *Per service*. The amount reimbursed by a payer to a provider for a service performed depends on many things including the network contract between the provider and the payer, the status of the provider as in-network or out-of-network, and the geographical location.

I. Claims Adjudication Formulas used by Payers

a) "Billed Charges" – "Excluded Expense" – "Discount Amount" = "Allowed Amount" (also known as "*Considered for Benefits*")

b) "Allowed Amount" – "Deductible" – "Coinsurance Amount" – "Copay Amount" – Coordination of Benefits Amount = Net Paid Amount

c) "Deductible" + "Coinsurance Amount" + "Copay Amount" = "Patient Responsibility"

These formulas clarify the **Explanation of Benefits (EOB)**, a document which the health plan sends to the member for each claim submitted by a provider.

Figure 08.1: Medical Claims Adjudication Formula

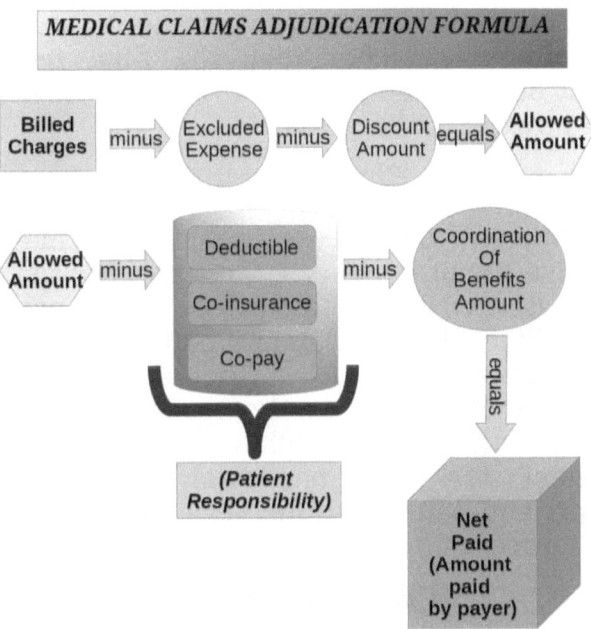

Billed Charges or Billed Amount

This is the charge billed by the provider for the service or procedure. This is almost never the amount that is finally paid and is usually way higher than the final reimbursement amount. This billed amount comes from a provider-maintained document known as a chargemaster.

Chargemaster

A *chargemaster* or charge description master is the comprehensive list of items (services, procedures, equipment, supplies, drugs, etc.) with their prices that a provider like a hospital can bill to a health plan or a patient.[24]

The chargemaster has prices that are several times the actual costs of the items and only serves as the starting point for negotiations with a health plan on what it will receive as reimbursement for that particular item. Unfortunately, uninsured patients can sometimes get slapped with bills for the full, inflated prices of items on the chargemaster.

Excluded Expense

Expense that is not covered by the health insurance policy – this is usually the responsibility of the member. The excluded expense does not include discounts, deductible, coinsurance, copay, or coordination of benefits.

Discount Amount

This is the discount negotiated by the health plan to the billed charge/price for the service/procedure or other item. For example, the hospital might have a billed facility-charge of $1,500 for a colonoscopy. But a particular health plan might have negotiated a discount of $500 – so, in this case, if the excluded expense is $0, the allowed amount would be $1,000. This allowed amount is what this particular health plan will pay this particular provider for this service. But the discounts negotiated with various providers are different. Thus, the allowed amount for the same service with different providers contracted with the same health plan might differ. A government health plan like Medicare usually pays much less for any service – in the case of a colonoscopy, the Medicare facility-charge allowed amount might only be about $760.

Allowed Amount

As explained above, this is the negotiated amount for the service that the provider will receive per the contract with the health plan. Allowed amounts for the same service might differ widely for different providers contracting with the same health plan – this is because providers vary in their negotiating power. A powerful and large health system in a geographical area will usually be able to negotiate better allowed rates with a plan than a smaller hospital or provider practice. The discount and the allowed amount are closely guarded secrets as part of the contract between the health plan and the provider. This contractual secrecy and variation in rates paid for services between providers are the main reasons why consumers/members are rarely able to get estimates, at the time they are receiving healthcare services, of what the costs for these services are. The costs are detailed out much later only when the medical bills and the Explanation of Benefits are generated. The Federal government has tried to address this secrecy in 2019 and 2020 through a series of price transparency initiatives.

Paid (Net Paid) Amount

This is what the health insurance company pays the provider for the claim. This is always less than or equal to the allowed amount (depending on what the patient responsibility is).

Sample Explanation of Benefits (EOB)

A sample EOB is shown below. Using the claims adjudication formula discussed previously, it is possible to understand the various components of the EOB. An EOB is sent to the member by the health plan for each claim it receives from a provider.

Figure 08.2: Sample Explanation of Benefits

Claim #: 91239945-01 (1) Patient #: 99523766 (3)
Patient: JANE DOE (2) Provider: ABC MEDICAL CENTER (4)

(5) Dates of Service	(6) Proc. Code	(7) Amount Billed	(8) Not Covered	(9) Remark Code	(10) Discount Amount	(11) Discount Code	(12) Allowed Amount	(13) Deductible Amount	(14) Co-pay Amount	(15) Covered Amount	(16) Paid At	(17) Payment Amount
01/18-01/18/2017	87086	$37.01	$0.00		$21.23	ECA	$15.78	$0.00	$0.00	$15.78	100%	$15.78
01/18-01/18/2017	87186	$84.00	$0.00		$69.47	ECA	$14.53	$0.00	$0.00	$14.53	100%	$14.53
01/18-01/18/2017	87088	$34.99	$0.00		$21.39	ECA	$13.60	$0.00	$0.00	$13.60	100%	$13.60
Column Totals (18)		$156.00			$112.09		$43.91	$0.00	$0.00	$43.91		$43.91

| | | | | | | | | Other Credits or Adjustments (20) | | | | $0.00 |
| Patient Responsibility (19) | $0.00 | | | | | | | Total Payment (21) | | | | $43.91 |

The claim number (1), patient/member name (2), patient ID (3), and provider name (4) are self-explanatory. The dates of service (5) for services/procedures carried out are shown as individual rows along with the medical billing codes (6) for the same. In some cases, a description of the service or procedure might also be provided. The EOB might be for an institutional/facility claim (generated by a hospital or other facility), or for an outpatient/professional services claim (generated by a physician-practice or an outpatient provider). Medical billing codes used are ICD-9 diagnosis codes, ICD-9 procedure codes, revenue codes, HCPCS (Healthcare Common Procedure Coding System) codes and CPT (Common Procedural Terminology) codes. Not all of these types of codes are found on all types of claims. Also, some EOBs provide just the descriptions for the services and not the codes. The billed amount (7) is the amount billed/charged by the provider – this usually comes from the previously described chargemaster. The discount amount (10) is the amount deducted from the billed amount to arrive at the allowed amount (12). If there are deductibles, co-pays, or co-insurance amounts, those are listed for each line item. Thus the payment amount (17), which represents what the health plan pays to the provider, is always less than or equal to the allowed amount (depending on what the patient responsibility – usually the sum of deductible, co-pay, and co-insurance amount is). The patient responsibility amount is also shown on the EOB. The EOB is not a bill. It does not require any action by the member who receives it. The bills for the patient-responsibility amounts are sent by the providers to the members directly.

It is important to understand that multiple claims (and hence EOBs) can be generated for a single episode of care. For example, if a woman gives birth to a baby in a hospital, one can expect to receive at least 4 different EOBs linked to 4 different claims: (1) The hospital's claim for inpatient services linked to the delivery; (2) The obstetrician's professional services claim; (3) The anesthesiologist's claim for professional services like epidural anesthesia that might have been given to the woman in labor; (4) The pediatrician's claim for professional services rendered for the newborn baby.

II. Types of Medical Claims: Professional and Institutional

The two main types of medical claims are *professional* and *institutional*.[25]

Institutional claims are submitted by institutional providers or facilities. They are for services, room-and-board, and other treatment provided by a healthcare institution. Institutional providers include hospitals, Skilled Nursing Facilities (SNFs), Hospice Organizations, Outpatient Physical Therapy/Occupational Therapy/Speech Pathology Services, Comprehensive Outpatient Rehabilitation Facilities (CORFs), End Stage Renal Disease (ESRD) providers, Home Health Agencies (HHAs), Community Mental Health Centers (CMHCs), Critical Access Hospitals (CAHs), Federally Qualified Health Centers (FQHCs), Histocompatibility Laboratories, Indian Health Service (IHS) Facilities, Organ Procurement Organizations, Religious Non-Medical Health Care Institutions (RNHCIs), and Rural Health Clinics (RHCs). Institutional claims are submitted electronically using the 837I (I stands for *Institutional*) file-specification or on paper using the CMS-1450 (UB-04) form. Important information that the institutional claim contains include:

(1) Diagnoses that the patient had, coded using ICD-10 diagnosis codes.

(2) Type of Bill, a 4-character code that identifies the type of facility (inpatient, outpatient, clinic, emergency room, etc.) and bill-type for the claim.

(3) Condition Codes, two-character codes to allow for submission of information about the patient, particular services, service venue and billing parameters which impact the processing of an institutional claim.

(4) Revenue Codes, 4-digit codes used for each of the multiple service/claim lines of the claim to identify the specific setting (hospital, emergency room, etc.) in which the service or procedure was performed.

(5) Services and procedures, coded using the Healthcare Common Procedure Coding System (HCPCS) codes and ICD-10 procedure codes. HCPCS Level I codes are the Common Procedural Terminology (CPT) codes owned by the American

Medical Association and describe medical procedures and professional services. HCPCS level II codes identify products, supplies, drugs, and services not included in the CPT codes. ICD-10 PCS (Procedure Coding System) codes are used for inpatient hospital procedures.

(6) Drugs and Medications administered, using National Drug Codes (NDC) – these are tied to the specific HCPCS codes used for "drug administration".

The claim also has information on the charged/billed amounts requested for payment.

Professional claims are bills submitted for services or procedures performed by physicians and other healthcare professionals. These professional services could have been performed in one of many healthcare settings: a hospital, a clinic, an outpatient surgery center, an emergency Room, a diagnostic laboratory, etc. Professional services claims are submitted electronically using the 837P (P stands for *Professional*) file-specification or on paper using the CMS-1500 form. Important information that the professional claim contains include:

(1) Diagnoses that the patient had, coded using ICD-10 diagnosis codes.

(2) Place of Service, a 2-digit code that identifies the organizational entity where services listed on the claim were delivered.

(3) Condition Codes, two-character codes to allow for submission of information about the patient, particular services, service venue and billing parameters which impact the processing of an institutional claim. On the professional claim, the condition codes are mostly used to indicate abortion services or workers' compensation claims.

(5) Services and procedures, coded using the Healthcare Common Procedure Coding System (HCPCS) codes and ICD-10 procedure codes. HCPCS Level I codes are the Common Procedural Terminology (CPT) codes owned by the American Medical Association and describe medical procedures and professional services. HCPCS level II codes identify products, supplies, drugs, and services not included in the CPT codes. ICD-10 PCS (Procedure Coding System) codes are used for inpatient hospital procedures.

(6) Drugs and Medications administered, using National Drug Codes (NDC) – these are tied to the specific HCPCS codes used for "drug administration".

Revenue codes are not used on professional claims.

If the physician or provider is an employee of a hospital or health system (and is a salaried employee), the professional services claim is submitted by the hospital on behalf of the physician. But the reimbursement from the health plan will not flow directly to the physician in this case. However, if the physician is an independently practicing physician who performs services in a hospital he/she has practice privileges in, the professional services claim is submitted by the physician's office and the reimbursement is also received directly by the physician.

III. Pharmacy Claims

Pharmacy Claims are submitted by retail pharmacies where prescriptions are filled. They are submitted using the NCPDP (National Council on Prescription Drug Programs) D.0 format. The claim can be submitted from a pharmacy to a health plan but can also be submitted from a pharmacy to a Pharmacy Benefit Manager. A Pharmacy Benefit Manager (PBM – explained later in this book) is an entity that employers, health plans,and others can contract with to manage the pharmacy and medication benefits of the members/employees. If an employer chooses to have pharmacy benefits be administered by a PBM, it is known as a *carve-out* of the pharmacy benefit. The pharmacy claim submitted has details of the drug, the NDC code for it, the dose, prescription, and the cost/charges billed. Inpatient medications administered during an episode like a hospital stay are not submitted using pharmacy claims – instead, they are submitted as part of the inpatient institutional claim.

IV. Diagnosis Related Groups (DRGs)

Instead of paying for hospital inpatient cases on a true fee-for-service basis, Medicare uses the Diagnosis Related Group system.[26]

This DRG system classifies all hospital inpatient diagnoses into about 400-500 groups. The idea is that diagnoses within a certain DRG are equivalent in terms of the cost-of-care provided in the hospital for that condition. Further adjustments based on factors like geography, wages in the area, and labor rate are used to calculate the reimbursement to the hospital for treating the patient. Thus, this system does not pay the hospital provider based on pure fee-for-service for procedures and services, and instead bundles various diagnoses into groups that are equivalent in terms of cost-of-care. Medicare calls this the Prospective Payment System (PPS). The DRG groups are further categorized into about 25 Major Diagnostic Categories (MDCs).[27]

Ambulatory Patient Groups (APGs) follow the same concept as DRGs, but are applicable to outpatient procedures.

Non-Medicare payers like Medicaid and private health plans also use DRGs, but the method of payment is not the same as that used by Medicare. In these cases, the DRG is simply used as a measure of output or the level of services provided.

V. Bundled Payment

Bundled payment[28] is a form of payment to providers where, instead of reimbursing each individual procedure or service performed for the patient (Fee-for-Service), the services are *aggregated* or *bundled* into an *episode of care* and the reimbursement is for the whole bundle or care-episode. These bundles usually include both hospital and post-hospital care. Surgical bundles are the most common, e.g., a bundle for knee replacement surgery might include the hospital stay, surgery, post-surgery follow-up visits, and rehab. The reimbursement amount for the bundle will cover the whole set of aggregated procedures and services that make up the episode of care.

Bundled payment can still be considered a form of Fee-for-Service reimbursement, except that the services are aggregated into a bundle that is paid as a whole.

VI. Relative Value Unit

Medicare and most private payers use the Relative Value Unit[29] (RVU) concept linked to the Resource-Based Relative Value Scale (RBRVS) system for reimbursing physician (professional) services. All physician services and procedures (which are coded using HCPCS codes) are assigned RVUs that are listed in the Centers for Medicaid and Medicare Services (CMS) Physician Schedule.[30] Specifically, there are physician work RVU, practice expense RVU, and malpractice expense RVU components. Using these components, along with the geographical practice cost index (specific to geographical locations in the US), and multiplying by the Medicare conversion factor for the year gives the final price that

Medicare will pay for the service or procedure. Private payers will usually pay more for the same service/procedure, but they also use RVUs to rate the financial value of the service. As an example, the 2020 physician work RVU for a *Gall Bladder Removal* is 17.48 while the work RVU for *New Patient Visit to an Outpatient Clinic* is 0.93. As is clear from the example, the RVU system favors surgeons, and physicians who perform a lot of procedures (proceduralists), over physicians who perform evaluation and management services for patients.

CAPITATION

Capitation is a payment methodology popular in managed care, where the health plan/managed care organization contracts with providers to provide health services to a group of members. For these services, the managed care plan pays the providers, provider group, or health system a capitated amount per member per coverage period e.g. $950 Per Member Per Month (PMPM) of coverage or $11,400 Per Member Per Year (PMPY). No Fee for Service billing is done by the providers in this situation. The providers are assuming the financial and clinical risk of taking care of this population of patients/members. If they can keep their cost of providing services to this population below the capitated amounts paid by the plan for the year, they will be able to pocket the difference as profit. On the other hand, in some cases, they might have to suffer losses if the cost of providing health services to the member population exceeds the capitation amount paid by the plan. The model described thus is called *global capitation*, which is meant to cover *all* healthcare services. There is another model, called *partial capitation* or *blended capitation*, where the capitation amount might only cover some types of healthcare services like preventive care and outpatient services, while the hospital and inpatient care is still reimbursed on a fee-for-service basis.

VALUE BASED REIMBURSEMENT/VALUE BASED CARE & POPULATION HEALTH

Value Based Reimbursement or Value Based Care is a healthcare payment methodology that aims to tie the quality (of clinical process and outcomes) and efficiency (cost of care) of clinical services to the reimbursement. This quality and efficiency together is considered the "value" of the care delivered. In other terms, value based care seeks to provide care that works towards achieving the previously described Triple Aim of healthcare.

Value-based care can be described in terms of a spectrum. This spectrum is based on the amount of financial risk that providers (rather than just payers) are willing to bear when they provide healthcare services for a population. In the value based care spectrum, the order of the "magnitude of financial risk" continuum is: Pay-for-performance (P4P) < Patient Centered Medical Home (PCMH) < Shared Savings < Bundled Payments < Shared Risk < Capitation (Full Risk) < Provider-sponsored Health Plans.

The first three categories in the value based care spectrum (P4P, PCMH, and Shared Savings) are what are known as "upside-only" risk. This means that the providers lose out on the bonus payments and incentives if they fail to meet the quality and efficiency targets, but suffer no penalties in financial terms. The last four categories in the value based care spectrum (Bundled Payments, Shared Risk, Capitation, and Provider-sponsored Health Plans) include "downside" risk. This means that the providers face financial penalties, and assume more of the financial risk that the cost of care could turn out to be too high, or higher than predicted or accounted for.

Pay-for-performance, as the term indicates, ties financial bonuses and incentives for providers to specific clinical quality and financial (lowering the cost of care) goals. The billing is done Fee-for-Service, but at the end of the measurement period, additional bonuses and incentives are paid out to the providers if they meet specific performance targets. There are usually no disincentives or penalties in this system for not achieving the performance targets.

A *Patient Centered Medical Home* is a team of healthcare providers like physicians, nurses, case managers, and medical assistants, who manage the healthcare needs and services for a particular member or patient population. The idea is that this improves the coordination of care required to better manage chronic conditions in the population. The reimbursement is usually Fee-for-Service (FFS) but the providers get paid additional amounts PMPM (Per Member Per Month) for care coordination and can also negotiate higher FFS rates.

Shared Savings programs reward providers with a

proportion of the savings achieved by reducing the healthcare expenditure of a population of members. The payer/health plan *shares* a part of the savings achieved in the cost-of-care with the providers who have taken care of the population.

Bundled payments based on episodes of care have been previously explained. Bundled payment models involve some downside risk for the providers if their costs run higher than the reimbursements offered for the episodes-of-care bundles.

Shared Risk programs are those in which the payer shares a part of the financial risk of the cost-of-care with the providers, while also sharing the savings from lowering the cost-of-care. Thus, there is true upside and downside risk being assumed by the providers who contract with a payer in a shared risk program.

Capitation models, which were described previously, are the next category in the continuum and represent significant downside risk for the providers.

The final category in the value based care continuum is that of *Provider-sponsored Health Plans*. These are health plans that are created by providers who care for the member population and also cover it (like a health plan). Thus, in this situation, the provider also becomes a payer and assumes significant financial risk for the healthcare costs of the population.

As described before, *Population Health Management* involves all the activities that need to be carried out to make a *Value Based Care* arrangement successful. There are 5 major parts to Population Health Management:

1. **Program Design, Network Contracting, and Financial Set-up** for the member population and the payer, employer, and provider entities that will enter into the agreement.

2. **Data Integration** (of both payer and provider data) in order to enable activities like care coordination and analytics that are required for effective population health.

3. **Analytics and Insights** generated about the member population from the integrated data.

4. **Care Management and Coordination** Activities.

5. **Stakeholder Engagement**, the stakeholders being the members, consumers/employers, payers, and providers involved.

In spite of a major push by the government and private payers towards value based care, adoption of risk-assuming (upside + downside) value-based-care by providers remains low. Upside-only value based reimbursement (VBR) has been more enthusiastically adopted by providers and up to 50% of their revenue comes from some sort of VBR contract. However, most providers are assuming downside financial risk in less than 10% of their VBR contracts. This is understandable, since Fee-for-Service billing and reimbursement has served providers and health systems well, and many of them see VBR as a race to the bottom.

PAYER-PROVIDER CONVERGENCE

Payer-provider convergence is the process underway where payers are buying up provider practices and health systems across the country and providers are assuming more financial risk and starting their own health insurance plans. Thus, payers are starting to take on provider characteristics and providers are beginning to act more like payers. Hence the convergence.

MEDICAL COST INFLATION AND WHY IT IS DIFFICULT TO CONTROL

Medical Cost Inflation is defined as the annual rate at which medical expenditures rise for the population. Medical cost inflation in the US has consistently trended much higher than the Consumer Price Index that measures regular inflation. For example, from 1965 to 2020, medical cost inflation has averaged more than 5.5% annually while the consumer price index (that tracks general inflation) has increased less than 4% annually in the same time period. One of the primary reasons, among many, for the high rate of medical cost inflation in the US is the "third-party payer" system based on health insurance. In this system, the consumer of healthcare services does not directly pay the price of these services to the provider. Instead, the consumer depends on the health insurance company to pay the provider. Thus, in this complicated transaction, there are 4 major players:

1) Member or consumer (patient).

2) Payer (health plan) or health insurance company (could be a government health plan).

3) Employer (healthcare insurance purchaser for employed individuals).

4) Provider (physician, hospital or other entity that delivers

healthcare services to the member).

It can be argued that at least 3 of these entities are either indifferent to keeping healthcare costs down or are actively interested in seeing healthcare costs rise!

The employer is the one entity of the four that is interested in controlling medical costs and keeping them from rising rapidly. This is because, at least in self-insured plans, the employer is contractually bound to pay medical claims submitted by providers for services delivered to employees who are members of the employer-sponsored health plan.

The member/consumer is indifferent to rising healthcare costs because he/she is only concerned about the annual premium. Since the provider is paid by the health insurance plan, the consumer does not feel the need to reduce healthcare utilization or find other ways to reduce medical costs like shopping around for the lowest price for a particular service or procedure. This is changing a bit because of high-deductible health plans and high co-pay and co-insurance rates on certain plans.

The providers, since they are engaged mostly in Fee-for-Service billing, are actually rewarded financially for both high per-unit billing and high utilization of services by the members.

The health plan or payer, who one might think has the most reason to control medical costs (since its profit is the revenue from insurance premiums minus the medical costs and administrative expenses), is also not very interested in controlling medical costs very strictly unless it is a government plan. Private plan payers, especially if they are corporate entities like private or public companies, are interested in increasing both revenue and profit (earnings) every year. A rise in revenue can be achieved in two ways – increasing the membership of the plan (quite difficult to achieve in a specific geographical area) or facilitating an increase in the insurance premiums. Thus, it is in the health plan's interest to let medical costs rise every year, since they can always raise member premiums to cover the costs of paying out medical claims. But in the bargain, they get to increase their absolute profits. For example, if a health insurance company collects $10 billion in premiums from 1 million members enrolled in fully-insured plans, pays out 80 percent of the amount (i.e. $8 billion) in medical cost claims, and spends another $1.7 billion as expenses, its profit is $300 million and the profit percentage is

3%. Next year, if the health plan is still aiming for a 3% profit margin, the only way to increase the absolute profit without increasing membership is to let the premium revenue (which is dependent on medical costs) rise. So, if healthcare costs are expected to rise 10%, and the health plan increases its premiums accordingly so that premium-revenue increases to $11 billion the next year, and 80% of that amount (i.e. $8.8 billion) is paid out in medical claims, with the same 17% expenses (i.e. $1.87 billion), the 3% profit now rises to $330 million – increase of $30 million over the previous year.

Also, if the health plan is mostly serving employers through self-insured plans (also called Administrative Services Only or ASO plans), it really has no interest in keeping medical costs very low.

That 80% number for medical costs as a percentage of revenue is not arbitrary. The Affordable Care Act of 2010 requires small group plans to have a medical loss/cost ratio (the percentage of premium revenue collected that is spent paying providers) *floor* (minimum) of 80% and large group plans to have a medical loss ratio *floor* of 85%. So, even if a small group plan is able to hold down medical costs to 75% of premium revenue, it will have to distribute the saved 5% back to the members and consumers as rebates. Thus, there is even more reason for a health plan to increase its absolute profit by increasing total revenue – since reducing medical costs does not work after a point in boosting earnings.

9. PAYER DATA

Payer data is of two major types:
1) The *medical and pharmacy claims data* submitted by providers for reimbursement.
2) *Data gathered for care management purposes* in specialized care management systems.
In addition, a third type of data is now being seen with payers: the clinical data from EMR systems that was discussed in chapter 4.

As discussed in chapter 4, payer data is wide but not rich. This is because it usually provides the full detail of all the healthcare services and procedures the patient/member has sought and received, but not in the sort of detail that exists in the clinical data repository of EMR systems maintained by providers.

MEDICAL AND PHARMACY CLAIMS DATA

As described in chapter 8, claims data includes details of the patient/member's diagnoses, procedures, facility of care, physician providing care, and other important information.

There are two main ways to understand the medical and pharmacy claims data that payers work with. One is to understand the file specifications for the HIPAA 5010 Electronic Data Interchange transactions dealing with claims submissions and payment. These include the previously discussed 837P, 837I, and pharmacy claims NCPDP specifications. However, it is much simpler to understand the details and components of medical and pharmacy claims data by studying the All Payer Claims Database (APCD) file-submission specifications of various US states. For example, the details of the Colorado APCD specs.[31]

Using these file-specification documents, one can understand that medical claims data contain elements like:
1. Member identification and eligibility data
2. Diagnoses
3. Services and Procedures, including revenue and procedure codes
4. Facility for treatment
5. Billing, Service, and Organizational Provider Information
6. Type of Bill and Place of Service

7. Billed and paid financial information from the claim
8. Drugs administered including codes

Pharmacy claims data contain elements like:
1. Member identification and eligibility data
2. Prescribed Drug
3. Dose, Route and other prescription information including drug codes
4. Pharmacy information
5. Charged and Paid Amounts as financial information
6. Prescribing physician information

CARE MANAGEMENT AND UTILIZATION MANAGEMENT DATA

As described in chapter 6, care management (case management and disease management) and utilization management processes generate data. The data generated by care management and utilization management processes include:
1. Nurse assessments
2. Patient self-assessments and surveys
3. Clinical measurements that might have been recorded by the patients/members
4. Medical review and prior authorization data.

These data are stored in care management systems that payers own and operate.

10. LIFE SCIENCE COMPANIES

Life science companies include pharmaceutical, biotechnology, medical device & technology, digital health, professional services, and clinical trials & research companies that are involved in creating and working with new treatment therapies and regimens.

Life science companies have to go through at least two very important processes for their financial survival. The first is to go through the process of approval of their drugs, therapies, or devices with governmental agencies. The second process is that of getting health insurance companies to cover the treatments and therapies that they have come up with. Both these processes are long, arduous, and involve sustained effort.

PHARMACEUTICAL COMPANIES

In the healthcare world, traditional pharmaceutical companies are involved in the discovery, creation, and production of drugs that are used as medications for treatment of diseases or as disease-prevention methodologies (like vaccines). Pharmaceutical companies are involved in intensive research and development operations in order to create new drugs and bring them to market. The pharmaceutical industry is highly regulated with regard to the process of creation, patenting, testing, and selling of drugs.

For every drug that they make, pharmaceutical companies evaluate demand, marketing costs, and competitors for establishing the *Wholesale Acquisition Cost* (WAC). This is the starting-point-of-negotiations price at which pharmaceutical wholesalers & distributors purchase these products. In a sense, this Wholesale Acquisition Cost is similar to the *Chargemaster* prices that are maintained by US hospitals and health systems. Discounts and rebates are usually applied to the WAC, based on market share, volume, prompt payment deals, and other factors.

Research Operations

Research operations in a pharmaceutical company involve 2 main components: Drug Discovery and Drug Development.

Drug Discovery

Drug discovery is the process of identifying potential drugs and chemical molecules which might prove effective in treating specific diseases or conditions. It involves understanding the changes in metabolic and chemical pathways within the body that take place in adverse medical conditions, and finding substances that can alter these pathways in a beneficial manner. Modern techniques like computer-aided molecular-modeling and simulations of molecular reactions have made it possible to screen huge numbers of molecules for identifying candidate medications.

Drug Development

Drug development comes into play after drug discovery is complete and a potential drug has been identified. The process of getting this drug to the stage of a medication that can be sold in the market as a treatment is a long one and involves determination of formulation and dose, safety testing, in-vitro and in-vivo study protocols, and clinical trials. *Contract Research Organizations (CROs)* and professional services organizations are often utilized by pharmaceutical companies for the process of drug development.

The whole Research and Development (R&D) process for drug discovery and development is long and arduous. In the US, it takes an average of 12 years for an experimental drug in a laboratory to reach the stage of being a medication that is sold in the market. And only 1 in 1000 experimental drugs reach the stage of human testing. Of the drugs that reach the human-testing stage, only 1 in 5 are approved as medications.

Despite modern advances, drug discovery is still time-consuming, and quite expensive. The total cost of development of a new drug could be in the billions of dollars.

Two main types of studies or trials are involved in the drug R&D process. The first are Clinical trials, which are usually Randomized Controlled Trials (RCTs). The second are Observational Studies or what is known as Real World Evidence (RWE).

Randomized Controlled Trials

Most drugs have to pass randomized controlled trials as part of the approval process. A Randomized Controlled Trial is the purest form of a medical experiment or clinical trial that aims to reduce or eliminate bias when evaluating new treatments. This is accomplished by random allocation of subjects to two or more groups, treating them differently, and then comparing the groups statistically with regard to a measurable response. In the usual two-groups model of an RCT, the experimental group receives the treatment or drug being evaluated, while the control group receives either no treatment or a placebo. The process of blinding is also used in order to further reduce sources of bias. A single blind study is one in which only the researcher performing the study knows which subjects are receiving the treatment and which are in the control group, as well as what treatments were given. In a double-blind study, neither the patients nor the researchers know which study group the subjects are in. In a triple-blind study, the subjects, researchers, and the people carrying out the statistical analysis do not know which treatment subjects received.

Observational Studies and Real World Evidence (RWE)

Observational studies draw inferences from a sample from a population where the independent variable is not under the control of the researchers - because of ethical concerns or logistical constraints. Observational studies, which are also referred to as studies to derive Real World Evidence (RWE), are often used for drugs *after* they have gone live in the market. They are used to evaluate the real-world performance of treatments. They are useful because of the following reasons: (1) Randomized Controlled Trials might not have the sample size and power to answer every single question about a treatment or drug (2) In some cases, ethical and logistical constraints make a randomized controlled trial impossible for a particular treatment modality (3) Widespread adoption of a treatment or drug might bring up uncommon adverse effects not observed during the randomized controlled trial.

Observational studies have the tendency to be affected by various biases in terms of the subjects and the effects. Many statistical techniques are available to reduce the bias-sources in observational studies, but they can never be as bias-free as randomized controlled trials. However, in situations where an RCT is not feasible or sufficient, observational studies provide valuable data and inferences.

Brand Name Medications

When a pharmaceutical company invests a lot in R&D to successfully create a new drug, it acquires a patent on it. This prevents peer-companies from copying the drug formulation and selling it as a competing product with the same chemical combination. Thus, the pharmaceutical company creates a brand name for the drug when it is first released to the market, and it uses its patent to ensure that the said brand name represents the only product that contains the medication. After a certain number of years, when the drug goes off-patent, other competing pharmaceutical companies are allowed to create their own products containing the drug (with their own brand names) and also permitted to create generic medications (which do not have any brand name). As an example, the drug atorvastatin (used to lower blood cholesterol levels in patients with heart disease) was developed by the pharmaceutical company Warner-Lambert (which was later acquired by the pharmaceutical company Pfizer) and sold under the brand name of Lipitor®.

Generic Medications

When a pharmaceutical company's drug goes off-patent, competing pharmaceutical companies are allowed to manufacture the drug and sell it under just the original drug/chemical name without the attached brand. This is known as the generic version of the drug. As an example, the drug atorvastatin sold under the brand name Lipitor® by Pfizer/Warner-Lambert went off-patent in the year 2011, after which significantly cheaper generic versions made by a number of other companies entered the market.

HEALTHCARE BIOTECHNOLOGY COMPANIES

The definition of a healthcare biotechnology company is not fully clear, but it broadly defined as a company that uses living organisms and their products (bacteria, fungi, enzymes, and even animals, etc.) to manufacture drugs and medications. The assumption is that the traditional pharmaceutical companies create drugs using just chemicals and artificial materials while biotechnology companies use living organisms and their products. However, this definition does not hold true any more since most pharmaceutical companies are also engaged in biotechnology and have huge biotechnology divisions. Healthcare Biotechnology companies might be involved in the production of small molecule chemical drugs like traditional pharmaceutical companies, but they are better known for producing what are known as *biopharmaceuticals* or *biologics*. Biologics can be produced in several ways: *extraction* from organisms, production using *recombinant DNA technology*, production in *tissue cultures* like is done for many vaccines, or production through *gene therapy*.

Biologics are usually complex organic molecules, much more complex that regular chemical drugs. When a company creates a new biologic, it usually applies for and receives a patent from the US government that gives it exclusivity for several years. Once a biologic goes off patent, other companies can produce versions of the biologic. *Biosimilars* are to biologics what *generics* are to regular medications. However, since biologics are very complex molecules, the approval process for producing a biosimilar is significantly more involved than that for producing a generic.

As an example, adalimumab, sold under the brand name Humira® by AbbVie, is a biologic used for the treatment of rheumatoid arthritis, ankylosing spondylitis, psoriasis, ulcerative colitis, and several other auto-immune conditions. It was approved in 2002 and went off patent in 2016. Adalimumab is a monoclonal antibody (the letters *mab* at the end of its name stand for monoclonal antibody) made using recombinant DNA technology. Biosimilars for adalimumab are now available in countries like India, but not yet in the US.

MEDICAL DEVICE, EQUIPMENT, AND TECHNOLOGY COMPANIES

These are companies that create and manufacture medical devices, equipment, and technology. A medical device is anything that is used for a medical purpose. It can be as simple as a thermometer, or complex like an implantable pacemaker, cardiac stent, or knee implant. Medical technology companies also make products like monitoring equipment, ventilators, and durable medical equipment that is used at home (e.g. CPAP machine for sleep apnea).

11. PHARMACEUTICAL DISTRIBUTORS/WHOLESALERS

Pharmaceutical Wholesalers and Distributors buy drugs from pharmaceutical manufacturers at the Wholesale Acquisition Cost (minus applied discounts and rebates) and sell them to pharmacies at the Wholesale Acquisition Cost (WAC) plus some negotiated percentage. They also enable discounts negotiated between manufacturers and other customers. The 3 largest pharmaceutical distributors in the US are McKesson, AmerisourceBergen, and Cardinal Health. Pharmaceutical distributors are true middlemen, in that they are not responsible for either the manufacture or the coverage of drugs for the health plan members. Their job is to be part of the supply chain for pharmaceutical products.

12. PHARMACIES

Pharmacies purchase drugs from pharmaceutical distributors (or in some cases directly from pharmaceutical manufacturers) and are responsible for their dispensing to patients. Pharmacies can be physical (independent, part of a retail chain, part of a grocery or other type of retail chain, etc.) or mail-order pharmacies. Pharmacies usually have warehouses in order to store the drugs they procure from the wholesalers or the manufacturers. In addition, there are specialty pharmacies that deal in complex, and usually expensive, products like biologics and self-injectable drugs. Mail order pharmacies have been growing in number. These do not have physical locations for dispensing drugs to patients, and instead send drugs through the mail. Many mail-order pharmacies are owned by Pharmacy Benefit Managers (PBMs) or by retail pharmacy chains.

13. PHARMACY BENEFIT MANAGERS (PBMS)

Pharmacy Benefit Managers (PBMs) are the most complex part of the pharmaceutical puzzle. PBMs usually do not work with the physical pharmaceutical products themselves and never handle drugs and dispensing. However, they are involved in managing prescription drug benefits for a large proportion of the US population and also process more than 60% of the prescriptions written. The largest PBM in the US used to be Express Scripts and CVS Health. However, both of these merged with health insurance companies in 2018. The health insurance company Cigna acquired Express Scripts and CVS Health acquired the health insurance company Aetna. In fact, this trend of health insurance companies merging with or creating/owning PBMs has accelerated. The largest US health insurance company UnitedHealth Group has its own PBM OptumRx, and also bought another PBM named Catamaran. Anthem, another large health insurance company, has a PBM named IngenioRx. And Humana has bought a PBM named Enclara. PBMs do carry out the basic pharmacy-claims administration tasks for health plans. But they are also involved in a very complex set of activities where they deal with private insurers and self-insured employers, pharmaceutical manufacturers, and pharmacies. PBMs carry out a lot of tasks under the prescription drug management umbrella. These include the following.

(1) Maintaining Pharmacy Networks: Similar to provider networks that are created and maintained by health plans, pharmacy networks comprise of pharmacies that have contracted to provide services to a particular health plan's members. It is the PBM that creates the network and negotiates the reimbursement rates and fees with the participating pharmacies.

(2) Operating Mail Order Pharmacies: Many mail-order pharmacy operations are owned by PBMs.

(3) Managing Formularies: A formulary is a list of drugs covered by a health plan. PBMs negotiate discounts with pharmaceutical manufacturers in return for getting their drugs on to formularies.

(4) Claims processing: Claims processing for pharmacy

claims.

(5) Pushing generics: Advocating and pushing for widespread adoption of generic medications rather than brand name drugs.

(6) Medication Therapy Management and other Care Management type programs: These are also delivered through PBMs.

(7) Negotiating rebates from pharmaceutical manufacturers: In exchange for inclusion on the formulary, PBMs negotiate rebates from pharmaceutical manufacturers. Part of these rebates are passed on to the health plan or employer sponsoring the coverage, but some are retained by the PBM.

The core value that PBMs bring to their clients, the private health insurers and the employer-sponsored plans, is the lowering of prices paid for pharmaceutical products. PBMs do this through 2 methods. The first is price negotiation with pharmacies (using the volume-power of all their payer and employer clients) to reduce the amount paid for drugs through *discounts*. The second is the *rebates* negotiated directly with drug manufacturers which apply after the drugs are sold. Manufacturers offer rebates to PBMs to get their specific drugs listed on a formulary and thus achieve sales volume. Thus, PBMs negotiate with both pharmacies and pharmaceutical manufacturers, for discounts and rebates respectively, in order to make lower drug prices available to their payer clients and their plan members.

PBMs have accused of not passing on all the rebates to their payer clients. However, this has changed in recent years and PBMs do pass on most of their rebates to the payer clients while charging a high up-front fee.

Another criticism has been that the rebates mechanism of PBMs actually encourages pharmaceutical manufacturers to mark up the list prices of their products in order to cover the rebate that will need to be paid to the PBM. "Spread pricing", is yet another issue. This refers to a maneuver in which the PBM charges the health plan client higher prices for generic drugs than it pays the pharmacies that it gets them from, and pockets the difference.

A lot of the payer and consumer issues with PBMs and the pharmaceutical sector in general are related to the lack of price transparency. This is similar to the situation in the core medical services sector, which also suffers from a lack of transparency in prices. Some recent executive orders by the US

White House have sought to impose price transparency on providers.

FIGURE 13.1: PHARMACEUTICAL SUPPLY CHAIN FLOW

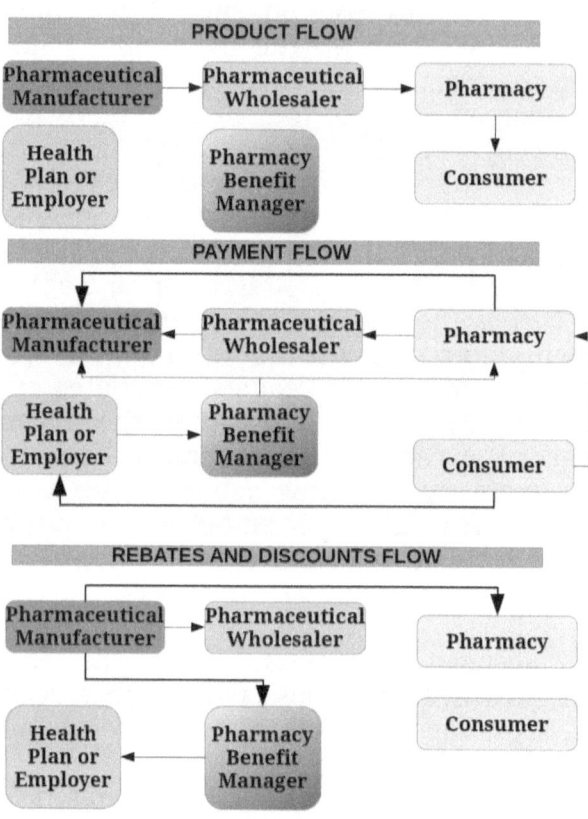

PHARMACEUTICAL PRODUCT PRICES

The concept of a *price* for a pharmaceutical product or drug is a not as clear as it should be. The *price* varies based on the entities involved in the buy-sell transaction, and their location. There are various concepts and definitions involved.[32][33]

Wholesale Acquisition Cost (WAC)

This is the baseline price at which pharmaceutical wholesalers purchase a product from a pharmaceutical manufacturer. This does not usually include discounts, rebates and other amounts applied.

Average Manufacturer Price (AMP)

This is the average price paid to a pharmaceutical manufacturer by pharmaceutical wholesalers for a drug distributed to retail pharmacies.

Average Sales Price (ASP)

The weighted average of all non-Federal sales by pharmaceutical manufacturers to pharmaceutical wholesalers applying the effects of charge-backs, discounts, rebates, and other modifications, whether it is paid to the wholesaler or the retailer.

Actual Acquisition Cost (AAC)

The price that retail pharmacies pay to purchase a drug from a pharmaceutical wholesaler. This is usually the Wholesale Acquisition Cost plus a markup (about 10-15% on branded drugs and greater on generics).

Estimated Acquisition Cost (EAC)

This is a state Medicaid program's best estimate of the price paid by retail pharmacies to wholesalers for a particular drug.

Maximum Allowable Cost (MAC)

Some private and government payers cap reimbursement for certain generic and multi-source brand products. The capped price for each drug is its Maximum Allowable Cost.

Siv Raman

Usual and Customary Price (U&C price)

The price of retail medications to consumers. This includes the cost of the drug (Actual Acquisition Cost) plus the pharmacy's markup. The pharmacy usually also receives a dispensing fee for every prescription.

14. THE GOVERNMENT ROLE IN HEALTHCARE

As briefly introduced in chapter 1, the US Federal Government role in healthcare is extensive. Even state governments play a major role in healthcare, both financially and through regulation. The US does not have a nationalized healthcare system, socialized medicine, or what is known as a *single payer* (the "single" payer being the government) system, unlike countries like Canada, the UK, and Italy. However, the US government spends huge amounts of money on healthcare every year. US National Healthcare Expenditures by type of service and source of funds are available on the website of US Centers for Medicare & Medicaid Services (CMS).[34] These clearly show how much the US Federal and State Governments spend on healthcare. For example, in 2018, the total spending on healthcare in the US was about $3.6 trillion. Of this, the US Federal Government's spending on Medicare was about $750 billion. The Federal Government spent about $370 billion on Medicaid, and state and local governments spent about $226 billion as well on Medicaid. The Federal Government spent about $17 billion on the CHIP program, and state and local governments spent another $1.4 billion. The Department of Defense (a Federal Government department) spent about $41 billion, and the Department of Veteran Affairs (another Federal department) spent about $78 billion. Thus, one could say that about half of all US healthcare is funded by the government.

Additionally, the US income-tax code exempts employer-paid premiums for health insurance from federal income and payroll taxes. Also, the portion of premiums employees pay is typically excluded from taxable income. This costs the US Federal Government about $270 billion annually in lost revenue and payroll taxes.

We are going to read a bit more about the largest government programs in healthcare: Medicare, Medicaid, and the CHIP program.

MEDICARE

Medicare[35] started in 1966 and is mainly a health insurance program for seniors age 65 and older. However, some younger persons with specific disabilities, and individuals with End Stage Renal Disease (ESRD) and Lou Gehrig's disease are also covered. Medicare taxes (payroll taxes) are deducted from all employee salaries in the US and the payment of these for at least 10 years is usually required to qualify for Medicare at 65. There are other qualifying criteria as well.

In 2018, there were about 60 million Medicare beneficiaries in the US. Medicare has 4 main parts: Part A, Part B, Part C, and Part D.

Medicare does have out-of-pocket costs for beneficiaries, including premiums, deductibles, co-insurance, and co-pays. These vary based on various factors like the income status of the individual, how many years Medicare taxes were paid, and others.

Medicare Part A

Medicare Part A covers hospital and hospice stays, i.e. inpatient medical care that require admission to a facility like a hospital. Medicare Part A can also pay for admission to a Skilled Nursing Facility for up to 100 days.

Medicare Part B

Medicare Part B is medical insurance that covers outpatient services like clinic visits, durable medical equipment, diagnostic tests, dialysis, and many others. There is a deductible for part B. After the deductible is met, part B covers 80% of the cost of services while 20% is the patient's responsibility. Many people on Medicare buy Medigap/Medicare Supplemental[36] policies from private insurers that help cover these 20% patient-responsibility payments.

Medicare Part C or Medicare Advantage

Medicare Part C allows Medicare beneficiaries to receive their benefits through capitated health insurance plans provided by private payers. In this case, the US Federal Government's *Center for Medicare and Medicaid Services* pays a capitated amount per beneficiary to the health insurance company, which then manages the benefits for this population of members who opt for Medicare Advantage Plans. A Medicare beneficiary who opts for Medicare Part C cannot claim benefits through parts A and B. Medicare Advantage plans are very popular since they usually provide a better and expanded set of benefits than those offered by Medicare parts A and B. Medicare Advantage plans usually offer services only within a defined provider network. Of the approximately 60 million Medicare beneficiaries in 2018, about 20 million were enrolled in Medicare Advantage plans.

There is a complex Medicare Risk Adjustment process by which the health insurance company that administers the Medicare Part C plan receives additional money (over and above the original capitated amount) in following years based on the updated financial risk profile of the member population. There is also a process by which CMS rates Medicare Advantage Plans on quality and performance every year using the Medicare Advantage Star Ratings.

Medicare Part D or Prescription Drug Plans

Medicare Part D started in 2006 and covers prescription drugs for beneficiaries. Any Medicare member with part A or B is eligible for part D and can enroll in a stand-alone Prescription Drug Plan. Also, Medicare Part C can offer integrated prescription drug benefits as part of MA-PD (Medicare Advantage with Prescription Drug Coverage) plans.

Medicare Cost Plans

Medicare Cost Plans are similar in some ways to Medicare Advantage plans. Those who enroll in Medicare Cost plans get to avail services within a specified provider network. But unlike Medicare Advantage plans, cost plans allow beneficiaries to go outside of the network, in which case the Medicare-covered services are paid for through parts A and B.

MEDICAID

Medicaid[37] started in 1965 as a health insurance program for low income individuals and those with limited resources. Medicaid is jointly funded by the US Federal government and the states. The federal government funds the states for a specified percentage of program expenses, called the Federal Medical Assistance Percentage (FMAP). States must ensure they can fund their share of Medicaid expenditures in their state Medicaid plan. State participation in Medicaid is actually voluntary, but all states are currently participating.

In a state, Medicaid might be delivered as a fee-for-service program or as a Medicaid Managed Care program. The former is similar to fee-for-service Medicare in terms of how providers are paid by the Medicaid program for services rendered to Medicare beneficiaries. Medicaid Managed Care, on the other hand, has the beneficiaries enrolled in a private health insurance plan which receives a capitated amount for the population from the state. In this sense, Medicaid Managed Care is a bit like Medicare Advantage. More than half the US states have some sort of Medicaid Managed Care program in place. Medicaid benefits and services differ from state to state. Also, some states bundle together Medicaid administration with other programs such as the Children's Health Insurance Program (CHIP). As of March 2020, about 64 million individuals were enrolled in Medicaid and about 6.7 million individuals were enrolled in CHIP.

The Affordable Care Act of 2010 expanded Medicaid eligibility to allow individuals with incomes of up to 133% of the Federal Poverty Level to qualify. Also, the law allowed for substantial Federal funding for the Medicaid expansion. However, as per a legal ruling by the US Supreme Court, the Medicaid expansion was not considered mandatory and was instead a choice that the states could make. About 10 states have opted not to expand Medicaid as part of the Affordable Care Act while the others have opted for the expansion[38].

Dual Eligibles

Dual eligibles[39] are individuals who qualify for both Medicare and Medicaid benefits coverage. In 2018, about 12.2 million individuals in the US were considered "duals". Medicare is the primary payer for most services, but Medicaid covers what is not covered by Medicare. Dual eligibles are usually in poorer health than other Medicare beneficiaries and also incur higher costs.

CHILDREN'S HEALTH INSURANCE PROGRAM (CHIP)

The CHIP[40] program covers uninsured children in families whose incomes are low but still too high to qualify for Medicaid coverage. About 6.7 million children were covered by

CHIP as of March 2020. As part of CHIP, the US Federal government gives matching funds to states for providing health insurance coverage to otherwise uninsured children.

15. REPORTING, ANALYTICS, AND OTHER DATA-RELATED HEALTHCARE OPERATIONS AND PROCESSES

There are several reporting, analytics, and other data-related processes and operations within healthcare, many of them connected to compliance activities. Some of them have been covered elsewhere in this book. Some other important ones are covered here.

CLINICAL MEASURES

Clinical measures[41] help track the quality of process and outcomes related to clinical services delivered by providers (both individual and institutional). Clinical measures can be reported using medical and pharmacy claims data, clinical data, or both. Many clinical measures are required to be reported annually by leveraging data captured in EHR systems. CMS requires some electronic clinical measures to be reported on annually by providers. Clinical measures are also obligatory as part of other clinical service and quality evaluation efforts such as HEDIS, Star ratings, Value Based Reimbursement contracts, etc. The Medicare Access and CHIP Reauthorization Act of 2015 (MACRA) utilizes clinical measures as part of its Merit Based Incentive Payments System (MIPS) and Alternative Payment Models (APMs).[42] In the simplest formulation, clinical measures consist of a denominator representing the individuals with the particular disease or condition, and a numerator that represents the individuals for whom a clinical quality guideline is correctly followed.

For example, one of the standard clinical recommendations for patients who suffer a heart attack (myocardial infarction) is to be given a beta-blocker drug for 6 months after the heart attack. A clinical measure to gauge the quality of care delivered by a provider for this guideline would be to include all patients with heart attacks in the denominator, and those who were put on beta blockers for 6 months in the numerator. The quality aim would be to achieve at least an 80% rate of compliance across all patients for this clinical measure.

FINANCIAL/EFFICIENCY MEASURES (COST OF

CARE)

Financial (also called efficiency or cost of care) measures are widely used by health plans to understand what the medical costs are for the insured population and what factors are driving them. Terms like costs Per Member per Month (PMPM) and Per Member per Year (PMPY) are used to understand how medical costs are trending. Also, these costs are broken down by type of utilization (inpatient vs outpatient), clinical care type (professional services, facility fees, medications), diagnoses, procedures, and so on.

A closely linked type of analytics/measures is actuarial analytics, which helps in predicting cost trends and financial risk for the future, and guides health insurance plans in setting premiums.

HEDIS REPORTING

The Healthcare Effectiveness Data and Information Set (HEDIS)[43] is a performance reporting framework that most health plans in the US follow and participate in. The HEDIS Performance Measures set is created and maintained by the National Committee for Quality Assurance (NCQA). Health plans participate in the HEDIS process every year. The process includes clinical measures using claims, clinical, and survey data, patient surveys, health plan measures, etc. NCQA publishes the Health Plan Ratings including HEDIS scores every year, using data gathered from the HEDIS Reporting process.[44]

CMS STAR RATINGS

CMS evaluates Medicare Part C (Medicare Advantage) and Medicare Part D (Prescription Drug) plans every year and assigns a 1-5 star rating to each[45]. The evaluation process includes a lot of quality and process reporting by the health plans. CMS Star measures cover 5 domains: Patient Experience, Outcomes, Intermediate Outcomes, Access, and Process. All Medicare Part C and Part D plans participate in the complicated Star ratings process each year.

POPULATION HEALTH MANAGEMENT REPORTING

Population Health Management reporting is done by plans and providers in value based reimbursement contracts e.g. Accountable Care Organizations or ACOs. This reporting involves quality measures (like clinical measures) and financial measures (like efficiency and cost of care).

PROVIDER AND NETWORK ANALYTICS

Provider and Network Analytics are tools used by health plans for evaluating the providers in their network in terms of clinical quality as well as financial efficiency.

CONSUMER ANALYTICS

Health plans use Consumer Analytics to better understand their members' experiences, healthcare needs, and quality/cost/access issues, and to stratify their member populations.

CLINICAL GROUPERS AND EPISODES OF CARE

Clinical Groupers are analytics software that help in constructing episodes of care from medical and pharmacy claims data. For example, medical claims from an elective surgery for knee replacement might be combined with rehabilitation visits and follow-up visits to create a single episode of care. These episodes of care are then used to evaluate quality and cost of care, as well as enable processes like the previously explained Bundled Payments.

RISK IDENTIFICATION AND STRATIFICATION

Risk *Identification*, in health plan parlance, refers to the process of assigning a financial risk/predicted medical cost score to each member and to the population as a whole. Then, based on the level of predicted financial risk, members are *stratified* into various risk categories. This process is closely linked to the previously discussed *Care Management*.

CARE GAPS/CARE OPPORTUNITIES

Clinical Care Gaps or Care Opportunities (also known as gaps in care) are identified shortcomings or lacunae in the clinical services and care provided to members. Care gaps can be identified for members through automated analytics, and also through manual surveys and assessments. Care managers are tasked with addressing these care gaps for the members. An example of a care gap is a missing mammogram for breast cancer screening for a woman aged 50-74.

PREDICTIVE MODELS/AI/MACHINE LEARNING

Predictive Models using Artificial Intelligence and Machine Learning are increasingly being utilized in healthcare to understand financial and clinical risk for members and patients, and to set clinical management goals for the population.

WHAT NEXT?

The rapid introduction to the US Healthcare system presented in this book should be able to get the reader started on a journey of self-exploration and self-improvement. What I recommend to learn more, in general and about specific topics, is not any particular book. Instead, it is best to utilize Internet search engines and find information on the web that explains topics of interest to the reader. I wish you the best on this voyage of discovery.

ABOUT THE AUTHOR

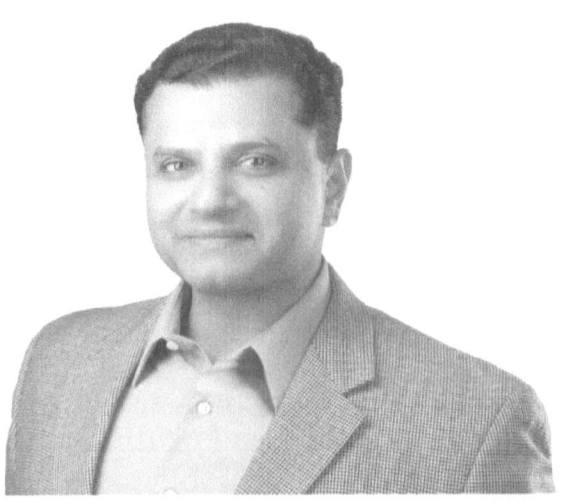

Sivakumaran "Siv" Raman is a physician who has spent most of his career in Medical Informatics and Analytics. With the experience of leadership positions at several large US health insurance companies, health systems, and information technology firms, he has extensive knowledge and expertise on the American healthcare system.

His previous book was *Just Enough R*, a freely downloadable primer on the R programming language, published on Smashwords.com and BarnesandNoble.com.[46]

Find Siv on Twitter:
@RamanSiv (https://twitter.com/ramansiv)

REFERENCES

1. American Health Care Spending;
https://www.crfb.org/papers/american-health-care-health-spending-and-federal-budget
2. Health and Social Assistance Sector Labor Statistics;
https://www.bls.gov/iag/tgs/iag62.htm
3. Bastiat's Broken Window Fallacy;
http://bastiat.org/en/twisatwins.html#SECTION_G002
4. Healthcare Expenditure 80-20 rule;
http://www.politifact.com/oregon/statements/2012/feb/23/alan-bates/does-20-percent-population-really-use-80-health-ca/
5. Healthcare Expenditure in the last few years of life;
https://www.ncbi.nlm.nih.gov/pmc/articles/PMC1361028/
6. Largest employer in every US state;
http://247wallst.com/special-report/2016/03/11/the-largest-employer-in-every-state/
7. Hospitals;
https://en.wikipedia.org/wiki/Hospital
8. PBMs According to the American Pharmacists' Association;
https://www.pharmacist.com/sites/default/files/files/Profile_26%20PBM%20Final%20071213.pdf
9. US taxpayers fund 64% of healthcare;
http://www.pnhp.org/news/2016/january/government-funds-nearly-two-thirds-of-us-health-care-costs-american-journal-of-pub
10. US BA+MD programs;
http://theperfectmed.com/programs.html
11. Nurse Practitioners;
https://en.wikipedia.org/wiki/Nurse_practitioner
12. Differential Diagnosis of Depression;
https://fpnotebook.com/psych/Depress/MjrDprsnDfrntlDgns.htm
13. US Independent Physicians;
http://www.beckershospitalreview.com/hospital-physician-relationships/20-key-insights-into-the-world-of-independent-physicians-33-of-us-physicians-are-independent.html
14. HITSP C-154;
http://www.hitsp.org/ConstructSet_Details.aspx?&PrefixAlpha=4&PrefixNumeric=154
15. EHR Adoption by Physicians in the US;

https://dashboard.healthit.gov/quickstats/pages/physician-ehr-adoption-trends.php

16. EHR Adoption by US Hospitals;
https://dashboard.healthit.gov/quickstats/pages/certified-electronic-health-record-technology-in-hospitals.php

17. The Healthcare Triple Aim;
http://www.ihi.org/Engage/Initiatives/TripleAim/Pages/default.aspx

18. HL7 Clinical Standards Organization;
http://www.hl7.org/index.cfm

19. US Health Insurance Coverage Statistics;
https://www.kff.org/other/state-indicator/total-population/?currentTimeframe=0&sortModel=%7B%22colId%22:%22Location%22,%22sort%22:%22asc%22%7D

20. Medical Necessity;
https://en.wikipedia.org/wiki/Medical_necessity

21. Case Management and Disease Management;
http://www.healthyinfo.com/tips/legal/diff.casemgmt.diseasemgmt.shtml

22. Federal Poverty Level;
https://www.healthcare.gov/glossary/federal-poverty-level-FPL/

23. Eight Main Methods of Heathcare Payment in the US;
https://www.acpjournals.org/doi/10.7326/M14-2784

24. The Healthcare Chargemaster;
https://en.wikipedia.org/wiki/Chargemaster

25. Healthcare billing claims: Professional and Institutional;
https://www.cms.gov/Outreach-and-Education/Medicare-Learning-Network-MLN/MLNProducts/MLN-Publications-Items/ICN006976

26. Diagnosis Related Groups;
https://en.wikipedia.org/wiki/Diagnosis-related_group

27. Major Diagnostic Categories;
https://en.wikipedia.org/wiki/Major_Diagnostic_Category

28. Bundled Payment;
https://en.wikipedia.org/wiki/Bundled_payment

29. Relative Value Units;
https://en.wikipedia.org/wiki/Relative_value_unit

30. CMS Physician Fee Schedule;
https://www.cms.gov/apps/physician-fee-schedule/search/search-criteria.aspx

31. Colorado All Payer Claims Database Specifications;
https://www.civhc.org/get-data/co-apcd-overview/

32. Avalere Health: Follow the Pill;
https://avalere.com/research/docs/Follow_the_Pill.pdf

33. Axene Health Partners: US Pharmaceutical Pricing;
https://axenehp.com/us-pharmaceutical-pricing-overview/

34. US National Healthcare Expenditures;
https://www.cms.gov/Research-Statistics-Data-and-Systems/
Statistics-Trends-and-Reports/NationalHealthExpendData/
NationalHealthAccountsHistorical

35. Medicare;
https://en.wikipedia.org/wiki/Medicare_(United_States)

36. Medigap and Medicare Supplemental Policies;
https://en.wikipedia.org/wiki/Medigap

37. Medicaid;
https://en.wikipedia.org/wiki/Medicaid

38. Affordable Care Act Medicaid Expansion status;
https://www.kff.org/medicaid/issue-brief/status-of-state-
medicaid-expansion-decisions-interactive-map/

39. Medicare Dual Eligibles;
https://en.wikipedia.org/wiki/Medicare_dual_eligible

40. Children's Health Insurance Program;
https://en.wikipedia.org/wiki/Children
%27s_Health_Insurance_Program

41. CMS Electronic Clinical Quality Measures;
https://www.cms.gov/Regulations-and-Guidance/Legislation/
EHRIncentivePrograms/ClinicalQualityMeasures

42. MIPS and MACRA;
https://www.cms.gov/Medicare/Quality-Initiatives-Patient-
Assessment-Instruments/Value-Based-Programs/MACRA-MIPS-
and-APMs/MACRA-MIPS-and-APMs

43. HEDIS;
https://en.wikipedia.org/wiki/
Healthcare_Effectiveness_Data_and_Information_Set

44. HEDIS NCQA Health Plan Ratings;
https://www.ncqa.org/hedis/reports-and-research/

45. CMS Star Ratings;
https://www.investopedia.com/terms/m/medicare-starrating-
system.asp

46. Just Enough R(Learn Data Analysis with R in a Day) by
Sivakumaran Raman;
https://www.smashwords.com/books/view/713592

INDEX

Alphabetical Index